The Promotion of Continence in Adult Nursing

David Colborn

The Nightingale Institute
Guy's Hospital
London, UK

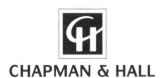

CHAPMAN & HALL

London · Glasgow · Weinheim · New York · Tokyo · Melbourne · Madras

113475502

Published by Chapman & Hall, 2–6 Boundary Row, London SE1 8HN, UK

Chapman & Hall, 2–6 Boundary Row, London SE1 8HN, UK

Blackie Academic & Professional, Wester Cleddens Road, Bishopbriggs, Glasgow G64 2NZ, UK

Chapman & Hall GmbH, Pappelallee 3, 69469 Weinheim, Germany

Chapman & Hall Inc., One Penn Plaza, 41st Floor, New York NY 10119, USA

Chapman & Hall Japan, Thomson Publishing Japan, Hirakawacho Nemoto Building, 6F, 1-7-11 Hirakawa-cho, Chiyoda-ku, Tokyo 102, Japan

Chapman & Hall Australia, Thomas Nelson Australia, 102 Dodds Street, South Melbourne, Victoria 3205, Australia

Chapman & Hall India, R. Seshadri, 32 Second Main Road, CIT East, Madras 600 035, India

Distributed in the USA and Canada by Singular Publishing Group Inc., 4284 41st Street, San Diego, California 92105

First edition 1994

© 1994 David Colborn

Typeset in 10/12 pt Palatino by Best-set Typesetter Ltd, Hong Kong
Printed in Great Britain by Page Bros, Norwich

ISBN   0 412 49460 4   1 56593 192 0 (USA)

A catalogue record for this book is available from the British Library

Library of Congress Catalog Card Number: 94-70261

∞ Printed on permanent acid-free text paper, manufactured in accordance with ANSI/NISO Z39.48-1992 and ANSI/NISO Z39.48-1984 (Permanence of Paper).

For Karen, M.B. and Big Jo

Contents

Preface

The prime motivation for this book has come from my experience with those who suffer from incontinence and from my contact, both in the clinical area and as a teacher, with those who care for them. Over the years I have developed a passionate interest in the subject and there is little doubt that in general terms the level of knowledge and awareness relating to the topic has increased. Despite this it is still apparent that continence promotion remains a somewhat fringe subject, both in practice and in theory. One of the difficulties which has become clear from discussion with nurses of all grades is that they feel that the only people who are capable of mastering the practicalities of continence promotion are full time continence advisers. It is unlikely that this view has stemmed from continence advisers themselves (those that I know are usually very grateful for all the help that they can get), or even from a reluctance on the part of nursing staff to develop their skills. The root of the difficulty appears to be a lack of awareness on the part of nurses of the skills that are required for continence promotion and also how they can be put into practice.

The aim of this book is to provide a reference text to enable all practising nurses to take an active part in continence promotion and the appropriate management of incontinence. In order to achieve this, a patient centred approach to care has been adopted focusing on the problems which the patients themselves are likely to complain of and which will be identified in the nursing assessment. In order to provide a foundation for this, relevant normal and disordered anatomy and physiology has been included, coupled with consideration of the potential psychological and sociological implications of incontinence. Overall the approach to care is a practical one and should not be difficult for the majority of nurses to adopt, since in reality continence promotion itself requires few skills which nurses do not already possess and also provides a field where, with a little application, nurses can become leaders. Having said this, it would be a mistake to assume that this book offers an exhaustive review of continence promotion. To claim this would be both arrogant and misleading. What this book does provide, however, is a basis for care and hopefully the inspiration for nurses to develop their own knowledge base in the subject and to seek further information as they require it.

ACKNOWLEDGEMENTS

This book could not have been conceived or completed without the help of a great many people. Of paramount importance have been the patients, carers, students and trained nurses with whom I have had contact over the years, and who have not only provided the clinical basis for the book, but also the inspiration and the impetus which I needed to write it. Mention must also be made of my colleagues at the Nightingale and Guy's College of Health who have tolerated my endless ranting on the subject and, in their own ways, provided me with a great deal of moral and practical support in terms of encouragement and source material. Particular thanks are due to John Hutton and Sarah Mobbs who dragged me kicking and screaming into the world of computers and word processing. Finally my thanks are due to Edward Loveless whose imaginative running of the ENB 978 course was a particular source of inspiration; to my mother, and to my wife, Karen, who have both helped me to maintain my belief that I could complete the book and have provided me with the support at home which has enabled me to do so.

David Colborn
London, UK
November, 1993

1

Defining the problem

THE ROLE OF THE NURSE IN CONTINENCE PROMOTION

Incontinence whether urinary, faecal or a combination of both is a problem which is encountered by all health care workers, especially nurses, at some stage in their careers. Because of this nurses have a wide range of experience of caring for incontinent people. But incontinence is still often seen as an intractable condition about which nothing can be done – except bombarding the sufferer with incontinence pads and other aids for containing the urine or faeces. If this fails, as frequently happens, the process of cleaning up must be embarked upon. There is little doubt that some nurses feel that, after a three year training, they have become proficient at wielding a mop and bucket to clean up incontinent episodes in record time before patients become wet or soil themselves again! This may appear to be a somewhat cynical comment on attitudes towards incontinence but it is undeniable that a large number of nurses still see incontinence as a problem which is time consuming, unexciting, singularly unromantic and certainly non-life threatening.

There is of course a degree of truth in this: all nurses have experienced the frustration of spending a long time washing a patient after an incontinent episode only to find that he or she is wet again within minutes. One study did in fact report that up to 80% of nursing time in a continuing care hospital for 200 elderly patients was spent in taking the patients to the toilet without them actually using it and clearing up after incontinent episodes (Southern and Henderson, 1990). When such data are considered, it is not unduly surprising that nurses do not feel inclined to take a great deal of interest in incontinence and are unable to adopt a positive attitude towards it. This is particularly sad as the tendency is to try to manage and contain incontinence rather than to initiate nursing interventions in order to reduce the number of incontinent episodes. In up to 70% of cases, patients could indeed be helped to regain full continence (DH, 1991). It could be argued that this approach falls into the category of cure as opposed to care and as such should be the domain of the doctors. Nurses, however, are the people most likely to identify the patients who are suffering from incontinence and will have the most contact with them in care situations. Furthermore, it is usually the choice of nursing intervention, as opposed to medical intervention, which results in patients experiencing an improvement in their condition and hence their quality of life. This is one of the most important considerations for nurses to grasp because without a realization of their crucial role in continence promotion they are in fact doing a disservice to their patients and, in many ways, to themselves. Not only are they failing to provide holistic care but, in addition, they will never experience the satisfaction of helping a patient to regain continence as a result of their efforts. Ideally of course a multidisciplinary approach needs to be adopted towards continence promotion in order to take into account the various factors which affect a person's continence status. It needs to be borne in mind, however, that this is an area where nurses can rapidly develop expertise and, by approaching the subject with a positive attitude, can take the lead in motivating other members of the team. It is for this reason that nurses should not only be aware of the problem of incontinence but should also see the promotion of continence as an integral part of their role, both as carers and as health educators.

THE ROLE OF THE CONTINENCE ADVISER

Although continence promotion needs to be considered by all nurses, there is still an obvious need for experts in the field who can act as 'resource persons' for their colleagues and provide advice and help when required. This is where the continence adviser can make a major contribution. Unfortunately there are only a limited number of continence advisers in post, making them a thinly spread resource. The exact duties undertaken by continence advisers vary across the country, being very much dependent upon what individiual health authorities or trusts have included in their role summary or job description. The majority of advisers have a responsibility to patients both in the community and hospital, and a large number of them have a background in district nursing. A district nursing qualification is required by some employers although it is arguable whether this really is an essential prerequisite. Most advisers have a caseload of patients, whom they see as necessary, and divide the rest of their time between out-patient clinics and teaching.

The creation of continence advisers' posts has only really happened in the last 10–15 years and in some cases their role has not been fully considered by the employing authority. Frequently the balance between the client caseload and time to carry out other activities such as research has been too heavily weighted towards the former, leaving continence advisers no time to assess the effectiveness of their role or to carry out their teaching commitments. The clinical grade of the advisers has also varied – ranging from staff nurse to senior nurse grades. This may not, in itself, be seen as terribly important by the individuals, although there are few people who would not prefer a higher grade and more money, but it does have a potential effect on who applies for the post and on how effectively applicants could carry it out. Part of the role of the continence adviser is to liaise with other staff in the health authority, particularly in supplies, and rightly or wrongly a bit of hierarchical muscle usually helps individuals to get their point across and have requests considered sympathetically. Such a situation is more likely to occur if a post is seen as being valued and is graded accordingly. It is essential therefore that anyone considering taking up a position as a continence adviser should ensure that the role is clearly defined and that any specialist knowledge and skills are recognized and rewarded.

DEFINING INCONTINENCE

Surely all nurses must know that individuals are incontinent if they have the misfortune to wet or soil themselves. This somewhat global approach, however, does not give any degree of measureability to the problem. If it were to be assumed as an accurate definition, it would probably include the majority of the population since there are few people who have not, at some stage in their adult lives, whether they would care to admit it or not, had what is best described as 'an accident'. Indeed one study of healthy female students in America found that at least 50% had wet themselves on at least one occasion (Wolin, 1969). This does not necessarily make them incontinent of urine, and there are many instances when accidents occur. One of the commonest is so called 'giggle' incontinence which occurs in young girls when they laugh, and which usually resolves after a comparatively short period of time without the need for any intervention. Then there are the times when toilet facilities have been unavailable for various reasons and when the toilet is finally in sight a small dribble of urine begins to leak from the urethra, or the times when the water is running into the washing up bowl or bath and the urge to pass urine is so strong that it may be impossible to prevent leakage, again usually only a small amount. Another fairly common experience is first thing in the morning during the period between sleep and waking when people need to pass urine and then proceed to dream that they are actually in the toilet and wake up to find that they are either on the verge of passing urine or have in fact already started to void in the bed. It is obvious that this is not incontinence but merely very rare incontinent episodes and it is for this reason that it is important to have a baseline definition from which to work in order to identify those who are truly incontinent.

What then is the definition of true incontinence? This is not necessarily an easy question to answer since a number of different definitions have been offered. The International Continence Society's definition states that incontinence is: '. . . a condition where involuntary loss of urine is a social or hygienic problem . . .' (Anderson *et al.*, 1988). This is a very patient centred definition and, although it is extremely valuable, it gives no real guidelines as to how frequently an individual is incontinent, or how much loss of urine or faeces needs to take place before a person can be considered to be suffering from true incontinence. While introducing measureability into a definition can lead to the risk of rigid application, it can be useful for planning care and setting goals with a patient and for subsequent evaluation of the effectiveness of that care. For this reason it is probably more helpful to consider a definition such as that offered by Thomas *et al.* (1980), who suggested that 'regular' incontinence could be considered as '. . . involuntary leakage or excretion of urine in inappropriate places or at inappropriate times twice or more a month, regardless of the quantity of urine lost.' This definition could equally well be applied to faecal incontinence.

Such an approach to incontinence automatically excludes all those who only have very infrequent incontinent episodes while, at the same time, giving a measureable baseline. In order for this definition to be patient/client centred, it needs to be used with a degree of flexibility. It must be recognized that there will be individuals who suffer only very occasional incontinent episodes, but who perceive these as a major problem which they require nursing intervention to help them overcome.

THE PREVALENCE AND COST OF INCONTINENCE

There are certain difficulties in obtaining accurate figures relating to how many people suffer from incontinence and how much this actually costs them as individuals and the health service as a whole. The main reason for this is that there is probably a large number of incontinent people who, for various reasons, choose not to seek any help for their problem and cope with it themselves with varying degrees of success. A related problem is the lack of recent large scale research on the subject. As a result of this many of the figures are somewhat dated and the majority of information relies on estimates which have been reached on the basis of comparatively small scale research projects and local interest.

One of the largest studies, involving over 20 000 people, was carried out by Thomas *et al.* (1980) who surveyed men and women over the age of 15 years on the lists of general practitioners and in the care of two London boroughs. The results of this study, which are summarized in Figure 1.1, suggested that overall 1% of men and 25% of women suffered from some degree of urinary incontinence. Despite the rigour of the experimental design and implementation, it is likely that these figures represent an underestimate of the true prevalence since they are based on the replies to a postal questionnaire and follow up interviews were restricted to a sample of those who had acknowledged that they suffered from incontinence rather that those who had replied that they never experienced incontinence. It is probably fair to assume that within this group there were a number of people who were not prepared to admit to having a problem of this nature. The research also considered how many people were actually known to the social service agencies involved in the study. The results of this element of the study cause some concern since they suggest that only a very small proportion of the people are actually known to the relevant agencies and therefore receiving help from them. The graph in Figure 1.1 shows the percentage of the respondents to the study who were incontinent of urine and also the percentage of the population known to be incontinent by the voluntary and statutory agencies.

Incontinence in hospitalized patients follows a slightly different trend to the figures relating to the community. Despite the impression (possibly brought about as a result of having to attend to the same patient more than once during a span of duty) which some nurses seem to have, that a very high percentage of their patients suffer from incontinence, the problem may be as low as 10% in general hospitals (Egan *et al.*, 1983). This figure compares quite well with the incidence of incontinence in the community as a whole. Other sources suggest, however, that the figure may be somewhat higher, particularly in continuing care settings such as nursing homes and long stay Care of the Elderly units where the incidence of urinary incontinence may be as high as 50% of residents (Mohide, 1986). These figures are of course averages; variations will occur, depending on the clinical specialty of the ward, the ages of the patients, nursing practices and other factors. They do give some indication of the extent of the problem, however, and current estimates suggest that there are over three million people in Britain who suffer from incontinence.

It is the supply of aids to help these people manage their incontinence which creates the greatest burden of direct cost to themselves and to the health service. The financial cost to individuals in terms of purchase of appliances is virtually impossible to estimate but, as figures related to the numbers of people known to social service agencies indicate (Figure 1.1), it is certain that a proportion of the people who are incontinent are buying their own aids to help them manage their problem with no assistance from health professionals. The cost to the NHS on the other hand is known to be comparatively large. Government estimates suggest that over £50 million per year

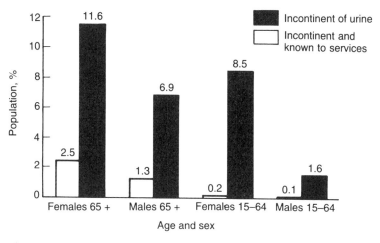

Figure 1.1 Prevalence of urinary incontinence (Thomas *et al.*, 1980).

are spent directly on pads and other appliances for the management of incontinence, and that in 1989 a further £18 million were spent on prescription items for the same purpose (DH, 1991). However, patients who have not undergone a thorough assessment in relation to their incontinence risk being provided with inappropriate pads which are more costly than necessary. Estimates by the Association for Continence Advice indicate that if assessment is carried out and appropriate action taken a reduction in cost of between 75% and 85% could be achieved (DH, 1991). Another factor in this equation which needs to be taken into consideration is the availability of a range of pads and appliances, dependent on the ordering policy of stores departments which in turn may be determined by regional contracts. The net result of this is that there is a limited range of products available to patients and care staff leading to inappropriate supply and use of aids. A continence adviser can play a central role, not only by recommending a suitable range of products based on their effectiveness rather than purely cost considerations, but also by giving a realistic indication of how many pads an individual may need over a given period rather than basing a person's supply on guesswork. This is a situation which can lead to stockpiling and misuse. It is not unknown to find pads being used as doormats, floor cloths, pet bedding, drawer liners and even towels.

ATTITUDES TOWARDS INCONTINENCE

Nurses' attitudes

As mentioned above some nurses' attitudes towards incontinence are far from positive and may well lead to unintentional, but none the less overt, mismanagement of patients. This in itself is unfortunate but worse still are the attitudes and approaches which actually lead to an increase in incontinence. Perhaps the most predominant of these is the belief that incontinence is an inevitable part of the ageing process and that older people can consider themselves lucky if they do not become incontinent at some stage in their later lives. This is certainly not a new idea and as far back as 1749 it was stated in *Synopsis Medicinae* that: 'Children or old people often piss a bed in their sleep, but these come not to the physician for a cure. It is a distemper very hard to be cured when it happens to those who are awake; in old persons it is altogether incurable unless hot baths relieve them . . .' (Allen, 1749). This was perhaps acceptable at the time of writing but it would appear that a not dissimilar attitude still exists some 250 years later despite the fact that we are meant to be living in a more enlightened age and have made considerable advances in the fields of medicine and nursing. Green (1986) suggested that it was ageist attitudes within the caring professions which were responsible for a large part of the problems encountered by the elderly in relation to incontinence and that these attitudes '. . . may lead to incontinence as well as to a failure to diagnose and treat it'. She also suggested that this attitudinal problem may be exacerbated by lack of education and stressed the need for greater teaching input on the subject in both pre- and post-basic nursing and medical training.

In 1983, the King's Fund recommended that medical and nursing schools (as they were then) should consider how the subject of incontinence should be dealt with in their curricula. This was prompted partly by the findings that, on average, medical students were only receiving 71 minutes of teaching input on the subject of urinary incontinence during their training and 21 minutes of teaching input on the subject of faecal incontinence (King's Fund, 1983). Figures for teaching time devoted to the subject during nurse training were not identified, although it was determined that any teaching which did occur was more likely to be associated with the management of incontinence as opposed to the promotion of continence. Many of the education managers who responded to their questionnaire felt that inadequate time was devoted to the subject as a whole. The lack of time devoted to this area in the curriculum, coupled with the fact that in most curricula any teaching about incontinence is included in relation to care of the elderly, has probably contributed greatly to the misconceptions which exist and also resulted partly in the association of incontinence with old age and any connotations which this may carry. Considering the numbers of people who suffer from incontinence and the fact that it is patently obvious that it is not an affliction which is restricted to the elderly it is remarkable that these attitudes still persist.

Another not uncommon response from nurses to patients who are incontinent is that of 'It's alright, it doesn't matter. We're used to it'. This is inappropriate for three main reasons. Firstly, it disregards the fact that being incontinent may matter very much to the individuals concerned and, in effect, it denies them the right to express their own feelings about it. Secondly, it may encourage patients not to try to control their incontinence. Thirdly, it could imply that the nursing staff themselves do not see incontinence as important and merely accept it as an inevitable occurrence, and are therefore less likely to attempt to take steps to prevent it from happening in the first place. These considerations aside, the statement is frequently belied by nurses' body language. It can be obvious to a patient that the nurse sees the incontinence as an imposition and would rather be doing something other than cleaning up the mess. This may lead the patient to be reluctant about informing the nursing staff when incontinence has occurred, with the result that he or she is left wet for long periods of time. Worse still, the patient may not even ask for toilet facilities in order to avoid disturbing the 'busy nurses' and will then suffer more frequent episodes of incontinence.

Carers' attitudes

It is also important to consider the attitudes of informal carers to incontinence since in the community setting they are the people most likely to be coping with a relative, usually a parent or spouse, who is experiencing a problem. For a large number of informal carers the onset of incontinence is the straw which breaks the camel's back. They are able to cope with most other aspects of the physical and psychological care which they have to give but the management of incontinence and the extra laundry and protection of furniture which is required when their relative (or significant other) becomes incontinent is too much of a burden. This is not unduly surprising since the level of information available to the general public is even more limited than that which is available within the caring professions, and the attitude that incontinence is intractable is almost universally held. This may lead to a degree of resignation and sometimes resentment since the mere fact that a relative is incontinent can lead to a dramatic curtailment of the person's social activities and normal lifestyle – not only because of the physical needs of the relative, but also as a result of perceived social stigma attached to the condition. This in turn may lead to a state of despair and, although incontinence is rarely identified as the prime reason for an individual's admission to hospital, in discussion with informal carers it often transpires that this was in fact the stimulus for them to seek help in the first place.

Attitudes of sufferers

Last but not least it is important to consider how the individual sufferer feels in relation to his or her incontinence. As mentioned above, there are some people who have developed their own management strategies to cope with incontinence and would find any intervention from health care professionals more of a disruption than a help. These people are, however, probably few and far between and it must always be borne in mind that a feeling of embarrassment may prompt individuals to minimize their problem and hence reduce the likelihood of their considering outside assistance. More often than not the attitude of people suffering from incontinence is very similar to that of a number of health care professionals and informal carers, in that it is a condition which they are expected to live with for the rest of their lives, and that little if any help is available other than the pads which they purchase themselves or have supplied by the general practitioner via the community nursing services. In some people there seems to be a high degree of denial associated with incontinence, again probably related to embarrassment and the feeling that nothing can be done.

It is feelings such as these which make the job of promoting continence particularly difficult. Part of the challenge for nursing staff is to overcome the hopelessness which is often associated with the condition, and to break through the barrier of embarrassment which may be present both in the patient and on the part of the nurse. In our society at least, excretion is considered a very private function and, although an everyday part of nursing care is to consider elimination needs and to take appropriate actions as necessary, it may still not be a topic which is aired and discussed with ease.

THE EFFECTS OF INCONTINENCE

Incontinence can have far reaching effects on an individual. These go beyond the physical problems which may be associated with it and, if holistic care is to be taken seriously as a concept, the social and psychological effects as well as the physical need to be considered. These all affect the quality of life which an individual experiences, and a major part of continence promotion must be seen as an attempt to improve this.

Physical problems

One of the greatest problems associated with incontinence is its effect on skin integrity. All of the major scales for assessing a person's risk of developing pressure sores (Norton and Exton-Smith, 1962; Waterlow, 1985; Pritchard, 1986) have recognized that if a person suffers from incontinence the chance of skin breakdown occuring is greatly increased. This results from two main factors. Firstly the presence of urine or faeces creates an abnormally moist environment which softens the epidermis and may lead to maceration and subsequent sore formation. Secondly the pH of urine and faeces differs from that of the skin, and both contain chemical substances which act as skin irritants leading to excoriation and painful rashes ('nappy rash'), again predisposing to breakdown. Another factor which needs to be considered in relation to this is the number of times that a person will need to be washed if he or she is incontinent. Frequent washing with soap and water removes the skin's natural oils with a consequent drying of the surface and an increased tendency for this to crack and break. This does not only lead to sores but also to an increased risk of infection which is unpleasant and painful for the individual, creates a need for increased nursing care, increases the cost factors and, in extreme cases, may lead to acute illness and death from septicaemia.

A less dramatic but equally unpleasant result of being incontinent is the fact that being in contact with damp or wet clothing is uncomfortable to say the least and can also lead to increased loss of body heat. This may be of particular importance in elderly or immobile people who are less able to control their temperature regulating mechanisms. Although this in itself is highly unlikely to result in the development of hypothermia it will certainly contribute to the discomfort experienced.

Social and psychological problems

It seems appropriate to consider these two areas together since they are inextricably linked and in the majority of cases have a profound impact on the lives of incontinence sufferers. Embarrassment has already been mentioned as a potential problem. One of the major elements of this is that involuntary loss of urine and faeces is associated with babies and childhood. For many sufferers the worry is that they are entering a period of second childhood and there may also be a fear that not only may other physical symptoms manifest themselves but that there may be some mental changes as well. This is of particular concern for the elderly who, as a result of lack of awareness and poor communication skills on the part of carers, are often patronized and spoken to as if they were children. In all age groups these fears can lead to a loss of self-esteem and subsequent withdrawal and depression, coupled with a degree of social isolation.

Isolation can also result directly from the physical manifestations of incontinence. The fear of not being able to reach a toilet in time, of wetting or soiling oneself in public and of odour problems are foremost in the minds of many incontinent people. As a result of this they will not attend social occasions and in some cases will not even leave the security of their own homes. Associated with this is the fear of possible rejection within a relationship and the risk of being seen as an object of ridicule especially since we live in a society which has a tendency to use humour, albeit cruelly at times, in order to cover up embarrassment. That is not to say that a certain amount of humour does not help when dealing with incontinence since, as with all areas of human existence, there is the potential for genuinely funny situations to arise. Having a sense of humour and keeping a balanced perspective can contribute to maintaining a positive and enthusiastic approach to the problems.

Other social considerations include, for example, the practicalities of increased amounts of washing, the need for more items of clothing to change into, the storage and disposal of pads and of course the burden of cost which all these entail.

At this point it is perhaps appropriate to include some comments from individuals who suffer from incontinence since in reality they are the only people who can really appreciate the true extent of the problem:

'I was taught pelvic floor exercises, but the importance was never stressed. I tried to do them for a while but I assumed that my incontinence was the result of having twins and that nothing further could be done about it.'

'I haven't dared to laugh too much since my last child was born.'

'When I started to wet myself I didn't want to tell anyone. I thought that they would think that I was a dirty old man.'

'I don't go out any more, I need the toilet every half hour you see and it's not easy when you are in public.'

'As a teenager I avoided women. Imagine the embarrassment of having a passionate fumble and her finding my underpants stuffed with loo paper!'

'We used to have a good sex life. Now we sleep in single beds.'

'When he became incontinent I just couldn't cope any more. I had to find a nursing home that was prepared to take him.'

The above are just a small selection of comments made by individuals and their carers who have been brave enough to seek help for their incontinence and have been able to discuss it freely and frankly with a continence adviser. But they are indicative of the detrimental effect which incontinence can have, not only on the lives of the sufferers themselves, but also on the lives of those around them.

The lack of knowledge relating to incontinence and the passive acceptance of it as an inevitable and intractable condition have certainly, in the past, presented a somewhat depressing picture. In a profession which is moving away from a history of traditional practices based solely on personal preference towards research based bractice, it is now essential that all nurses equip themselves with the knowledge and skills which are required to provide quality care and health education for their patients. The field of continence promotion should be no exception. Only by adopting a positive approach can this be achieved and the emphasis of care must be that rather than trying to determine how a person's incontinence may best be managed, the first thought should be how can the individual best be helped to become continent again. Only when this has been attempted should management of the incontinence be considered. In this way many people will be helped back to continence and those who do not become fully continent will be able to manage their incontinence appropriately, with a consequent improvement in the quality of their lives and those of the people around them.

REFERENCES AND FURTHER READING

Allen, J. (1749) *Synopsis Medicinae*, London.
Anderson, J., Abrams, P., Blairas, J. and Stanton, S. (1988) The standardisation of terminology of lower urinary tract function. *Scandinavian Journal of Urology and Nephrology* (Supplement), **114**, 5–19.
Department of Health (1991) *Agenda for Action on Continence Services*, HMSO, London.
Egan, M., Plymat, K., Thomas, T. and Meade, T. (1983) Incontinence in patients in two District General Hospitals. *Nursing Times*, **79**(5), 22–3.
Green, M. (1986) Old people and disorders of continence, in *Incontinence and its Management* (ed D. Mandelstam), Croom Helm, Beckenham.

King's Fund (1983) *Action on Incontinence*, King's Fund, London.

Mohide, E. (1986) The prevalence and scope of urinary incontinence. *Clinics in Geriatric Medicine*, **2**(4), 639–55.

Norton, D. and Exton-Smith, A. (1962) *An Investigation of Geriatric Nursing Problems in Hospital*, National Corporation for the Care of Old People, London.

Pritchard, V. (1986) Pressure sores: a risk assessment card. *Nursing Times*, **82**(8), 59–61.

Southern, D. and Henderson, P. (1990) Tackling incontinence. *Nursing Times*, **86**(10), 36–8.

Thomas, T., Plymat, K., Blannin, J. and Meade, T. (1980) Prevalence of urinary incontinence. *British Medical Journal*, **281**, 1243–5.

Waterlow, J. (1985) Pressure sores: calculating the risk. *Nursing Times*, **81**(48), 49–55.

Wolin, L. (1969) Stress incontinence in young healthy nulliparous female subjects. *Journal of Urology*, **101**, 545–9.

2

Urine production and the physiology of micturition

In order to understand fully urinary incontinence and the factors which may pre-dispose to it or even be direct causes of it, it is important to have a basic understanding of the normal anatomy and physiology of the urinary tract, the process of urine production and factors which may affect it and the physiology of bladder emptying. Although the majority of nurses will have had some teaching about the urinary tract during their training, knowledge can become somewhat rusty. Therefore this chapter includes what could be considered to be basic information as well as more advanced content. No apology is made for this since it is an attempt to provide a comprehensive picture rather than to make assumptions about people's previous knowledge.

ANATOMY OF THE URINARY TRACT

The urinary tract consists of the following components:

- two kidneys
- two ureters
- bladder
- urethra.

The kidneys

The kidneys are situated between the peritoneum and the posterior wall of the abdominal cavity (i.e. they are retroperitoneal). They lie above the waist and are protected to some degree by the eleventh and twelfth ribs, with the right kidney

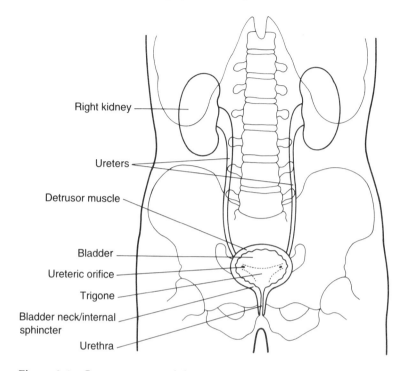

Figure 2.1 Gross anatomy of the urinary system (anterior view).

being slightly lower than the left because of the comparatively large area taken up by the liver. In adults each kidney is approximately 11 cm long, 6 cm wide and 2–3 cm thick, and is surrounded by three layers of tissue with differing functions. The innermost layer is the renal capsule, a term sometimes used to describe all three layers collectively. This consists of a smooth membrane in close contact with the surface of the kidney and serves predominantly to provide a barrier to infection. The middle layer of tissue is the fatty or adipose layer which again has a protective function in that it helps to cushion the kidney and also to hold it in place in the abdomen in conjunction with the outer layer, the renal fascia, which is a thin layer of fibrous tissue anchoring the kidney to the adjacent organs and the abdominal wall.

The blood supply to each kidney is provided by the renal arteries which enter the kidney at a point on the concave

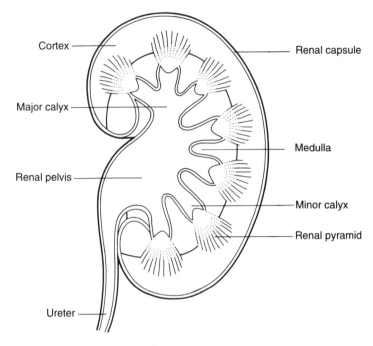

Figure 2.2 Cross-section of a kidney.

border called the hilus which also serves as the exit point for the renal vein which returns the blood to the inferior vena cava.

In cross-section the kidney can be seen to be made up of various distinct areas (Figure 2.2).

Lying immediately below the renal capsule is the cortex of the kidney which extends around and, at certain points, known as the renal columns, protrudes into the central region of the kidney called the medulla. This is where the collecting tubules of the kidney can be found. These appear as triangular or pyramidal structures (the renal pyramids) which have their bases pointing towards the cortical area and their points draining into cuplike structures (the minor calyces) which in turn drain into larger cups (the major calyces). On average there are approximately 15 renal pyramids per kidney, each with an accompanying minor calyx and two or three major calyces

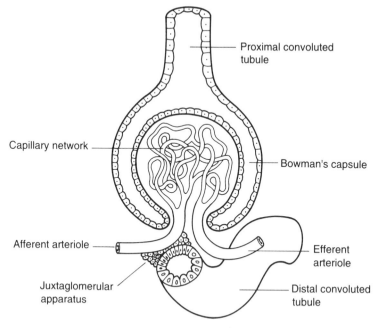

Figure 2.3   Cross-section of a glomerulus.

which finally open out into the pelvis of the kidney which then drains into the ureter.

The nephron

The nephron can be considered to be the functional unit of the kidney where urine production takes place. There are approximately one million nephrons per kidney and they make up the bulk of its mass. Structurally a nephron (Figure 2.3) consists of a capillary network called a glomerulus which is surrounded by the Bowman's capsule where filtrate is collected.

These structures can be found predominantly in the cortex of the kidney. The Bowman's capsule then drains into a collecting tube, the proximal convoluted tubule, which in turn enters the Loop of Henlé which dips down towards the centre of the kidney and then returns to join the distal convoluted tubule (Figure 2.4). This then drains into a collecting duct which leads

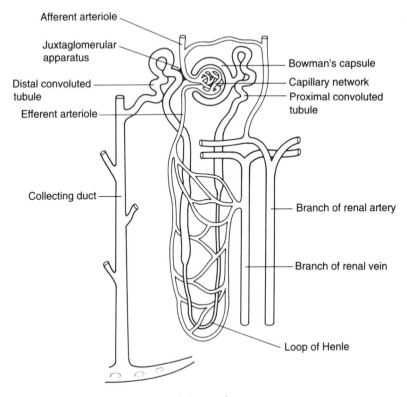

Figure 2.4   Gross structure of the nephron.

to the minor calyx. The combination of tubules and collecting ducts comprise the medullary region of the kidney.

The ureters

Each ureter is approximately 28 cm long extending from the kidneys through the retroperitoneal space and entering the bladder at the base through the rear wall. They consist of three layers of tissue and an inner layer of mucosa (which secretes mucus in order to protect the underlying cells from the variable pH of the urine) surrounded by a middle layer of longitudinal and circular smooth muscle and an outer coat. By peristaltic movements, the middle layer of muscle squeezes the urine which is draining from the renal pelvis down towards the bladder. The outer coat is a fibrous one which extends into the bladder wall and serves to anchor the ureters in place. At the point where they enter the bladder there is no true sphincter mechanism and urine is prevented from flowing back up them as a result of folds in the bladder muscle, the angle at which they are inserted and the downward pressure exerted by the bladder (during the filling phase and whilst contraction is occurring) at the point where they pass under its lower surface.

The bladder

This is situated in the lower part of the pelvic cavity just behind the symphysis pubis bone. In men the rectum lies behind the bladder whilst in women the vagina separates the rectum from the bladder and under normal circumstances the uterus curves anteriorly over it. Structurally the bladder consists of four layers of tissue. The innermost layer consists of mucous membrane and serves to provide protection for the underlying cells in a similar way to that of the ureters. This inner layer is folded into rugae. The next layer acts as a connective layer between the mucosa and the third layer which is the bladder muscle – the detrusor muscle. This itself consists of a sandwich of circular muscle between two layers of longitudinal muscle. The outer layer of the bladder only covers the upper surface and is made up from peritoneum. In the lower posterior wall of the bladder is an area known as the trigone, because of its triangular shape, which contains a large number of stretch receptors which transmit sensory impulses as the bladder fills.

The urethra

At the base of the bladder is the bladder neck which funnels down into the urethra. The anatomy of this differs between males and females. Males having an 's' shaped urethra which is 18–22 cm in length (Figure 2.5), whilst females have a straight urethra which is only 3–5 cm long (Figure 2.6). In the male, the first 2–3 cm of the urethra, the prostatic urethra, are surrounded by the prostate gland, the anatomy of which will be covered in Chapter 6. Immediately below this and sited on the

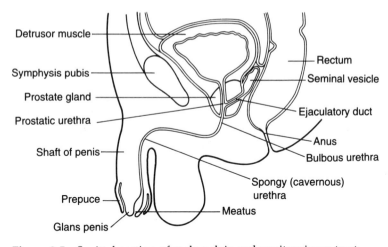

Figure 2.5   Sagittal section of male pelvis and genitourinary tract.

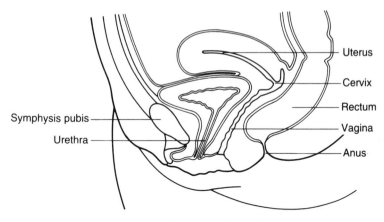

Figure 2.6   Sagittal section of female pelvis and urinary organs.

ventral surface of the male urethra is the veru montanum, a slightly raised mound of tissue, on which is the utriculus masculinus which is considered to be a vestigial uterus.

Associated with the bladder neck and the urethra are the urinary sphincter mechanisms. The first of these sphincter mechanisms is to be found at the bladder neck itself and consists of smooth muscle. In the male this is arranged as a circular band of muscle which is effective in achieving complete closure of the urethra. In the female the muscle fibres are inserted longitudinally into the wall of the urethra and are unlikely, in themselves, to be capable of causing closure by active contraction, although under normal circumstances the bladder neck will not open until detrusor contraction occurs. The next sphincter mechanism, the external sphincter, is the combination of smooth and striated muscle fibres which, in the male, can be found directly below the veru montanum and in the female, are arranged in a circular fashion and inserted for almost the whole length of the urethra (Gosling, 1984; Williams, 1989). Further urethral closure is achieved by the action of the pelvic floor muscles. The structure of the walls of the urethra differs slightly between the sexes. In the male there are only two layers of tissue: a mucous layer which is continuous with the mucous lining of the bladder and an outer submucous layer which connects the urethra to the surrounding tissues. In the female there are three layers: the inner mucous layer which is continuous with the external mucous layer of the vulva, an intermediate layer and an outer muscular layer arranged as described above.

THE PHYSIOLOGY OF URINE PRODUCTION

The production of urine involves a three stage process:

- filtration
- reabsorption
- secretion.

Filtration

This is carried out in the glomerulus which, as previously mentioned, is a capillary network contained within the Bowman's capsule. This network is supplied with blood from the afferent arteriole which originates from the renal artery itself (Figure 2.4). The whole of the filtration process depends predominantly on the pressure of blood entering through this artery which serves to force water and solutes contained in the blood through pores in the membranes of the glomerulus and into the cup formed by the Bowman's capsule. Although filtration is primarily dependent upon blood pressure various other forces come into play at this point which act against it. Firstly, there is the pressure exerted by the walls of the Bowman's capsule and the filtrate already present within it. Secondly, there is the osmotic pressure of the blood still remaining in the capillary network. Under normal circumstances the total positive pressure exerted is approximately 10 mm Hg which results in a filtrate volume at this stage of about 120 ml per minute, or 180 litres per day. Obviously this amount is not lost as urine and the vast majority of it is returned to the circulating blood volume by the next stage of the process, reabsorption.

Reabsorption

This takes place in the tubules which make up the remaining part of the nephron and is the result of both active and passive processes. Once the filtrate enters the proximal convoluted tubule approximately 80% of the water is reabsorbed as the result of osmosis. This is partly due to the active reabsorption of sodium ions from the proximal tubule which creates a high osmotic pressure in the tissues and blood vessels which surround it with the consequence that water is reabsorbed. This relatively high concentration of positively charged sodium ions is also responsible for the reabsorption of negatively charged chloride ions as the result of electrostatic attraction. Another substance which is thought to be transported actively is glucose. This is probably achieved by carrier enzymes in the membranes of the tubules and it is likely that these are limited in number resulting in a maximum amount of glucose which can be reabsorbed (the renal threshold or tubular maximum) which accounts for the presence of glucose in the urine of patients with diabetes mellitus. The filtrate then passes into the loop of Henlé where a comparatively complex mechanism involving transport of chloride ions out of the filtrate ensures that the osmotic pressure of the filtrate is low when it finally reaches the distal convoluted tubule and the collecting duct. It is at this point that anti-diuretic hormone (ADH), produced in the hypothalamus and stored and released by the posterior lobe of the pituitary gland, has an effect on the permeability of the walls of the distal tubule. In the absence of ADH the walls of the tubule and the collecting duct are virtually impermeable to water and no further water is reabsorbed, which results in dilute urine being produced. Conversely if ADH is being secreted water reabsorption is enhanced and the urine becomes more concentrated. The stimulus for ADH secretion is the osmotic pressure of the blood which is detected by osmoreceptors in the hypothalamus.

Secretion

This takes place in the tubules and is primarily a mechanism for controlling the pH of the blood and maintaining homeostasis. This is achieved by secretion of H^+ and ammonium ions into the tubule with a consequent raising of the blood pH. This is necessary because an average diet contains more acid producing foods than alkali producing foods and if this mechanism were not present the blood pH would be consistently too low. Other substances which are secreted into the tubules are potassium ions, creatinine and certain drugs such as penicillin.

The end product of these three processes is urine which drains from the kidneys into the ureters where it is forced towards the bladder by peristaltic contractions.

FACTORS AFFECTING URINE PRODUCTION

In health and under normal levels of hydration the body produces on average approximately 1–2 litres of urine per day (i.e. 1–1.5 ml per minute). The majority of urine production over a 24 hour period takes place during waking hours with only 20–30% of urine being produced during sleep (Wilson, 1990). Various factors may affect the rate of urine production in health, however, the three major ones are:

- fluid intake
- blood pressure
- temperature.

Fluid intake

Under normal circumstances fluid intake is controlled by the sensation of thirst. This sensation occurs when the body is approaching a negative fluid balance (although it is said that humans are the only animals which drink when they are not actually thirsty). When fluid loss is higher than fluid intake one of the first signs is that of a dry mouth which is interpreted by the brain as a sensation of thirst. Coupled with this the concentration of solutes in the blood increases which stimulates the hypothalamic thirst centre and causes a desire to drink which, if heeded, will result in a return to homeostasis. If this does not occur dehydration results and consequently there is decreased urine production and any urine which is produced becomes more concentrated. This is due in part to the drop in blood pressure resulting from a lower circulating volume which in turn causes a reduced glomerular filtration rate.

Excessive fluid intake which causes the body to be in a state of positive fluid balance results in an increase in circulatory volume with a consequent increase in glomerular filtration rate and the production of large volumes of dilute urine.

Blood pressure

It has already been mentioned that urine production can be affected by changes in blood pressure which result in a greater or lesser pressure within the glomerular capillaries. This, however, is accompanied by changes which occur as a result of specialized cells formed from the middle layer of the afferent arteriole known as the juxtaglomerular cells or juxtaglomerular apparatus. These cells are extremely sensitive to changes in blood pressure and are responsible for initiating the renin-angiotensin pathway. When the pressure of blood in the afferent arteriole falls below normal levels the enzyme renin is secreted into the plasma by the juxtaglomerular apparatus. The renin acts on angiotensinogen, a substance which is synthesized in the liver, to convert it to angiotensin I which in turn is converted to angiotensin II in the lungs. Angiotensin II stimulates the adrenal cortex to produce aldosterone which serves to increase sodium and water reabsorption in the distal convoluted tubules thus increasing the circulatory volume and a return to normal blood pressure at which time renin production is stopped (Figure 2.7).

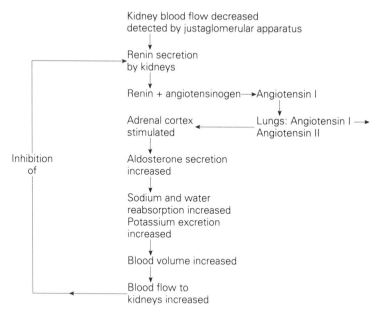

Figure 2.7   Renin-angiotensin pathway.

Temperature

When the temperature of the body is increased, either as a result of internal factors (e.g. fever) or simply as the result of a rise in the ambient temperature of the environment, dilatation occurs in the superficial vessels of the skin and fluid is lost as a result of sweat production. This creates a not dissimilar situation to that which occurs in mild dehydration and results in thirst and secretion of ADH, the action of which has been described above. A further response to a rise in temperature is constriction of the major abdominal vessels, including the renal arteries, which leads to a decreased blood supply to the kidneys, reduced filtration rate and also a reduced pressure in the afferent arteriole which may trigger the renin-angiotensin mechanism and hence lead to further water reabsorption. In situations where the ambient temperature is lowered, the superficial vessels constrict and the abdominal vessels dilate with the result that more blood passes through the renal arteries and the glomerular filtration rate increases with a subsequent increase in urine production.

THE PHYSIOLOGY OF MICTURITION

The ability to control bladder emptying is a process which is learnt, usually in early childhood, as the result of 'potty training'. Babies are incapable of exercising any control over this process and bladder emptying is dependent upon the action of a reflex arc. As the bladder fills the distension is detected by the stretch receptors in the trigone. At this point sensory impulses are generated and transmitted via the autonomic nervous system to the sacral area of the spinal cord (S2–S4) where the reflex arc is stimulated. Motor impulses return from the spinal cord again via the autonomic nervous system and initiate relaxation of the internal sphincter and contraction of the detrusor muscle with the result that urine is expelled (Figure 2.8).

Other than the voluntary control of the pelvic floor muscles this is an entirely involuntary process and further development of the nervous system is necessary before continence can be learnt and achieved. Voluntary control of micturition is dependent on the transfer of the sensory impulses from the bladder to the cerebral micturition control centre via the spinal cord tracts. Once an awareness of the need to void and also the social desirability of controlling voiding have developed, as the result of biological maturation and socialization, micturition becomes a controlled process as the result of nerve impulses from the micturition control centre which are transmitted down the spinal cord and serve to block the reflex arc (Figure 2.9). Although there is some controversy regarding the age at which potty training should take place, and some people claim to have trained their babies at a very early age, it is unlikely that successful control will be achieved below the age of 2 years.

For the majority of the time the control of micturition is an unconscious process, unless the bladder is overdistended to the point of discomfort, and when the need to void is felt the individual will find an appropriate place to pass urine and, once there, will allow the bladder to empty. One further element in the voluntary control of micturition is the relaxation of the pelvic floor muscles, which must be relaxed for mic-

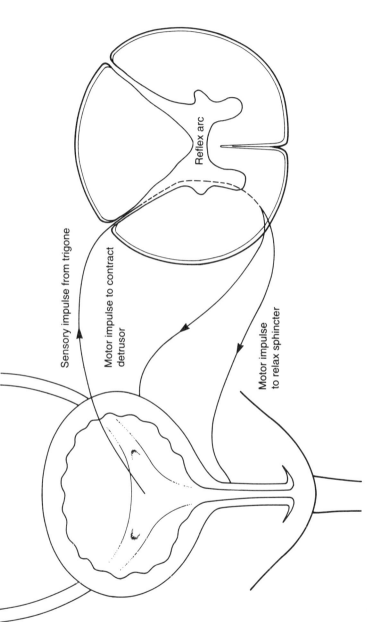

Sensory impulse from trigone

Motor impulse to contract detrusor

Reflex arc

Motor impulse to relax sphincter

Figure 2.8 Sacral reflex arc.

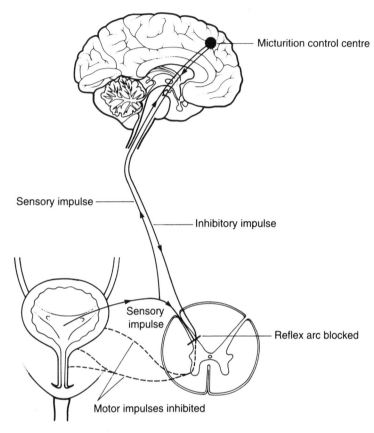

Micturition control centre

Sensory impulse

Inhibitory impulse

Sensory
impulse

Reflex arc blocked

Motor impulses inhibited

Figure 2.9   Inhibition of sacral reflex arc.

turition to take place. This combination of involuntary and
voluntary control over bladder emptying not only maintains
continence but, in the vast majority of people, also allows them
to empty their bladders at will regardless of the amount of
urine present. This skill is particularly useful if the oppor-
tunities to void are limited as the result of external constraints,
on long journeys with irregular availability of toilet facilities for
example. Average bladder capacity before discomfort is experienced is approximately 300 ml, although most people would
choose to void prior to this. Under normal circumstances, therefore, adults will void at intervals of 4–6 hours during the day
and should have no need to void during the night.

It is of course difficult to be 100% specific about what constitutes a normal pattern of micturition since individuals may differ quite considerably in their habits and needs. This fact should be borne in mind when assessing individuals in relation to their continence. The need to adopt an individualized approach to caring for people with incontinence cannot be over emphasized.

THE EFFECTS OF AGEING ON THE BLADDER AND MICTURITION

Although it must be stressed that incontinence should not be regarded as an inevitable problem of ageing, or a problem which is restricted to the elderly, it is important to recognize that there are certain aspects of the normal ageing process which may have a direct influence on an older person's ability to maintain continence.

Changes in kidney function

Urine production is, as mentioned above, largely dependent on the ability of the kidney to carry out the processes of filtration, reabsorption and secretion. In younger people this process is carried out very efficiently with only about one third of urine production taking place during sleeping hours, minimizing the need to void during this time and allowing for maximum rest. This level of efficiency decreases as people age, up to the point where the rate of urine production is almost constant over the 24 hour period. The consequence of this is that the elderly are much more likely to suffer disturbed sleep patterns due to the need to void during the night, a factor which may under certain circumstances also lead to nocturnal enuresis even if an individual is fully continent during the day. This will be discussed further in later chapters.

Bladder changes

Changes to the detrusor muscle differ little from those which occur in other muscles in relation to ageing. The muscle becomes less elastic, less efficient in its contraction, may suffer a degree of hypertrophy and in some cases will also have diverticula present, all of which will serve to decrease the efficiency of bladder function and may pre-dispose to the development of atonic bladder, incomplete emptying and incontinence.

Urethral changes

Prostatic hypertrophy, albeit not strictly a change in the structure of the urethra, is perhaps the most common change associated with the urinary system in ageing men and will be discussed in detail in Chapter 6.

In women the major anatomical change which takes place as a result of the ageing process is hormone-related. Postmenopausally, oestrogen levels begin to fall, although in many women no significant changes take place for several years if at all. If, however, a woman is affected by the fall in oestrogen levels various changes may take place. Firstly the walls of the urethra become less flexible and lose the pronounced folds which are present when normal oestrogen levels prevail (Figure 2.10); and thus the urethra ceases to possess as efficient a seal as previously. Secondly lack of oestrogen may result in an over sensitive trigone and urethritis which will cause similar problems to those experienced in cystitis or urinary tract infection. Coupled with this the woman may experience a degree of vaginitis with an inflamed vagina and vulva which is more prone to infection and ulceration. This condition is known as

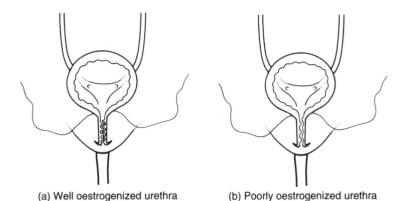

(a) Well oestrogenized urethra   (b) Poorly oestrogenized urethra

Figure 2.10 Urethral changes resulting from oestrogen deficiency.

atrophic vaginitis or sometimes less charitably, bearing in mind that women in their fifties may suffer from the problem, senile vaginitis. Further discussion of this problem can be found in Chapter 4. A final change which occurs, again partially associated with a fall in oestrogen levels, is that shrinkage and contraction of the vulval and vaginal tissues may cause the urethral orifice to migrate backwards so that it is actually within the vagina and can be found on its anterior wall. This is one of the reasons why it is sometimes extremely difficult to locate the urethral meatus in elderly women when attempting catheterization.

Nervous system changes

It is well recognized that the ageing nervous system is less well able to respond rapidly to internal and external stimuli. This is particularly significant in relation to the control of bladder emptying, and it is common for elderly people to experience little or no warning of the need to void as a result of reduced sensory output from the trigone and a delayed relaying of the message to the cerebral cortex which is further exacerbated by a delayed inhibitory impulse reaching the reflex arc. This is likely to lead to problems of urgency which, if not recognized and addressed, may lead to incontinence.

Although there are various other factors, such as reduced mobility and altered mental states, which may be associated with the ageing process and the ability to maintain continence, they are not exclusive to the elderly and will be discussed as appropriate.

In real terms it is not necessary to have an in-depth knowledge of the urinary system in order to promote continence. What is important, however, is that nurses have a sufficiently comprehensive grasp of the normal functioning of the system to be able to identify dysfunction, and thus instigate appropriate nursing interventions in order to try to correct this.

REFERENCES AND FURTHER READING

Blandy, J. (1989) *Lecture Notes on Urology*, 4th edn, Blackwell Scientific Publications, Oxford.
Cull, P. (ed.) (1989) *The Sourcebook of Medical Illustration*, Parthenon, New Jersey.

Gosling, J. (1984) The anatomy of the bladder and urethra, in *Urodynamics: Principles, Practice and Application* (eds A. Munday *et al.*), Churchill Livingstone, Edinburgh.

Guyton, A. (1990) *Textbook of Medical Physiology*, 8th edn, W.B. Saunders, Philadelphia. Chapter 19.

Hinchliff, S. and Montague, S. (eds) (1988) *Physiology for Nursing Practice*, Baillière Tindall, London. Chapter 5.

Tortora, G. and Anagnostakos, N. (1990) *Principles of Anatomy and Physiology*, 6th edn, Harper and Row, London. Chapter 26.

Williams, P. (ed) (1989) *Grays Anatomy*, 37th edn, Churchill Livingstone, Edinburgh.

Wilson, J. (1990) *Ross and Wilson: Anatomy and Physiology in Health and Illness*, 7th edn, Churchill Livingstone, Edinburgh.

3

Asessment of the individual

THE IMPORTANCE OF ASSESSMENT

Assessment is recognized as being of prime importance for the planning of appropriate nursing care and the subsequent nursing intervention (Roper, Logan and Tierney, 1990). Despite the recognition of this and the fact that elimination is included as part of a patient's general assessment, specific assessment related to a person's continence is frequently ignored, even if it is identified that a person has problems with the maintenance of continence. This may be due in part to the attitudinal problems which exist in relation to incontinence (see Chapter 1). Regardless of the reason for this apparent apathy, it cannot be stressed too greatly that appropriate assessment is absolutely essential if a person's incontinence is to be approached in a meaningful and positive manner; it is only by carrying out a full assessment that the individual patient's problems can be identified and the cause of the incontinence treated.

MULTIDISCIPLINARY INVOLVEMENT

One of the accusations which has been levelled against the development and implementation of nursing models and the nursing process approach to care delivery is that there has been an over emphasis on the nursing role in patient care to the exclusion of other disciplines. Although it has to be recognized that each discipline may have a discrete and specialist input in relation to caring for the patient, the principle of using a multidisciplinary approach to care should never be ignored, particularly in the field of continence promotion. Under ideal circumstances this co-operative team approach should be adopted at the stage of patient assessment and, in order to ensure continiuty of approach, in the delivery of care. Despite this ideal it must be recognized that there will be occasions, either as a result of unavailability of other staff or at worst lack of co-operation from colleagues in other disciplines, that the nursing assessment of a person in relation to his or her continence status may be the most detailed one that is performed or possibly the only one! Because of this the first part of this chapter will be devoted to the nursing assessment of the individual although this will also include suggestions as to when it may be more appropriate to ensure that other disciplines are involved with the patient.

THE ASSESSMENT PROCESS

As with all forms of patient assessment, the assessment of an individual in relation to his or her continence/incontinence relies on building a relationship of trust between nurse and client (Brown, 1988). This relationship is particularly important for the incontinent person since there is considerable social stigma attached to the problem and it may have taken great courage for the individual to acknowledge that he or she has a problem in the first place. Perhaps more sensitive still is the patient whose incontinence has been 'discovered' whilst undergoing treatment for an unrelated condition. In either case there is potential for embarrassment on the part of the patient and the nurse, a barrier which must be overcome if a therapeutic relationship is to be developed and a meaningful assessment carried out.

There are various measures which can be taken, as in the case of all assessments, to minimize the risk of poor communication between nurse and patient. Although these may be self-evident to the majority of nurses it is appropriate to re-emphasize them at this point.

Environment

The majority of patient assessments in the hospital setting take place in the ward at the patient's bedside. This is unlikely to be an ideal setting and it is difficult to encourage a person to talk about their most intimate details under these circumstances. It is particularly important to ensure privacy when discussing a problem such as incontinence, in order to put the client at ease (Campbell *et al.*, 1985). This is less likely to present difficulties in a clinic or health centre setting where nurses may have their own examination/treatment room but it is an important factor to bear in mind when assessing clients in their own homes since they may not have shared the fact that they are incontinent with their partners or family. The principle of confidentiality is still applicable in this setting.

Time

Time appears to be a commodity which is generally in short supply for nursing staff both in the institutional setting and in the community. Despite this it is essential that sufficient time be allowed for the initial assessment of patients since this is when they will form their first impression of the nursing staff and the foundations of the relationship will be laid. Time is also important to ensure that patients have the opportunity to express themselves without feeling that they are being rushed (Faulkner, 1992).

Terminology

Medical terminology may, at the best of times, be difficult for the lay person to understand. It has to be remembered that, although the use of professional terminology is second nature to nursing staff, many patients do not understand even what appear to be comparatively simple questions and explanations with regard to their conditions (Kagan, Evans and Kay, 1986). This problem is compounded in the field of incontinence since it is not only a difficult topic to discuss freely with a stranger, a fact which may make it more difficult for the patient to question what is being said, but there are also a myriad of terms in colloquial usage to describe both bladder and bowel functions. Many of these are so commonplace as to be almost universally understood but, as is usually the case with children, a large number of people have their own 'pet' words and phrases which they use to describe their excretory functions. Not only may these words be unfamiliar to the nurse but patients may also be reluctant to share them for fear of exposing a lack of knowledge or being judged on their use of language. This is an area where nurses need to be particularly sensitive and aware not only of the fact that some patients may use words that are wholly individual to them but also that there are regional variations in language usage and phraseology. Under these circumstances it is primarily the responsibility of the nurse carrying out the assessment to ensure, as far as possible, that both he or she and the patient are using terminology which is understandable by both parties. Any terminology which other staff may have difficulty in understanding should be noted on the assessment form so as to avoid possible confusion at a later stage.

INITIAL ASSESSMENT OF PHYSICAL ASPECTS

This constitutes the most important part of the nursing assessment, although it should not be performed to the exclusion of the other elements of the assessment process. If carried out effectively it is, in many cases, sufficient to provide the nurse with adequate information to implement a basic plan of care.

Time interval between voiding

As explained in Chapter 2 the adult bladder will normally hold approximately 300 ml of urine before a strong urge to void is experienced. The rate at which this volume is reached is variable and dependent on the rate of urine production but, unless there is an exceptionally large fluid intake or a person is dehydrated, it can be assumed for all practical purposes that urine is produced at a rate of between 1–2 ml per minute. At this rate of production it can be seen that voiding will take place at 3–6 hourly intervals. If voiding is more frequent than seven times whilst awake (Hilton and Stanton, 1981), and there are no factors which can be identified as being causative, then a person can be considered as having frequency (which will be discussed in Chapter 4). Infrequent voiding may be suggestive of disturbed sensory pathways from the bladder to the spinal cord (a problem which will be addressed in Chapter 6).

The only accurate way of determining the above is the use of a continence chart to record each time the person voids. Coupled with this there should be a record on the chart of whether this was an incontinent episode and, if not, whether the voiding was prompted by a member of the care staff or initiated by a request from the patient. This is the simplest use of a continence chart. However, it is also important to maintain a record of when the patient is dry since only by doing this can a detailed picture be built up of exactly when incontinence occurs. Use of such a chart will enable the nurse to determine whether or not patients have a pattern to their incontinence and what times of day it occurs. Ideally the chart needs to be maintained for a period of 7–10 days and should cover the whole 24 hour period. This should present few difficulties in an institutional setting where care staff are available during the night, but may present greater problems in the community if the patient lives alone or with informal carers. In reality there is no reason why patients themselves, or their carers, should not fill the chart in if they are able to; and if it is impossible to keep a record at night a record of when incontinence occurs during the day is better than no record at all!

One of the difficulties which may be encountered in either a hospital or a home situation is 'gaps' in the record as a result of people not remembering to check the patient and not completing the chart. This may occur for a number of very good reasons but it must be stressed to nurses and other carers that this record not only provides the information which is required to determine whether there is a pattern to a person's incontinence, but also a baseline from which any improvement or deterioration can be measured. This is why the importance of an accurate record cannot be over emphasized.

The information obtained from a chart such as this will give a comparatively comprehensive picture of a person's needs in relation to voiding. If, however, the chart is not being filled in correctly it may be beneficial to keep a more simple record since it is possible that asking for less information on a chart may encourage greater compliance with completion (Faulkner, 1992). Bearing in mind that it is the recognition of a pattern which is of prime importance the simplest chart which will yield useful information is one which records when a person is wet and when dry (Figure 3.1). This form of chart will give the minimum information which is required to commence appropriate nursing interventions for the patient.

Volume of urine voided

This is an additional piece of information which, although not as important as the interval between voiding, is nonetheless

CLIENT NAME:
* Use the following abbrevations   W = Wet   D = Dry   T = Used toilet
* Enter exact time as necessary

TIME	DATE												
01:00													
02:00													
03:00													
04:00													
05:00													
06:00													
07:00													
08:00													
09:00													
10:00													
11:00													
12:00													
13:00													
14:00													
15:00													
16:00													
17:00													
18:00													
19:00													
20:00													
21:00													
22:00													
23:00													
00:00													

Figure 3.1 Wet/dry chart.

extremely useful in leading to the identification of patient problems, the cause of their incontinence and, most importantly, if there is a need to manage the incontinence by the use of pads, which pads to recommend. Measurement of the volume of urine voided may present some difficulties especially if the patient is never able to void into a bedpan, urinal or commode. If the exact volume passed is considered to be of particular importance it is necessary to provide the patient with pads which are weighed prior to wearing and after each incontinent episode. Since one litre of urine weighs approximately one kilogram (i.e. 1 ml weighs 1 mg) it is possible by using this method to obtain fairly accurate measurements of the amounts of urine lost. It is somewhat time consuming, however, and may only be appropriate in an institutional setting with access to accurate scales. For the majority of patients it is sufficient to obtain approximate volumes of urine lost and make a judgement on the basis of experience. This judgement can be improved by taking the time to wet unworn pads (and, if necessary, bedding) with a measured volume of water in order to obtain an idea of how wet a certain amount of fluid will actually make a pad or bedding feel and appear. This will help to minimize the degree of subjectivity when estimating how much urine a person has voided and also the use of terms such as 'swimming in it' which, although descriptive and giving some indication that a large volume of urine is involved, are not helpful when attempting to draw up an objective record.

If it is possible to measure the urine in a more orthodox manner this is of course desirable and will give more accurate records. Volume of urine lost does not require a separate chart and can be included on either the simplified wet/dry chart or the continence chart as can be seen in Figure 3.2.

A further piece of information which is of great help when considering both interval between voiding and the volume of urine passed is that of fluid intake. This is almost invariably assessed and recorded for patients who are in an acute stage of an illness, but is frequently ignored when a person's continence status is being assessed despite its almost self-evident relevance. This again can be included on a single chart for use either by care staff or by patients themselves, and it may be possible to identify times when incontinence occurs which can be directly linked to the volume of fluid consumed. It is also

CLIENT NAME:
* Use the following abbrevations   W = Wet   D = Dry   T = Used toilet
* Enter exact time as necessary

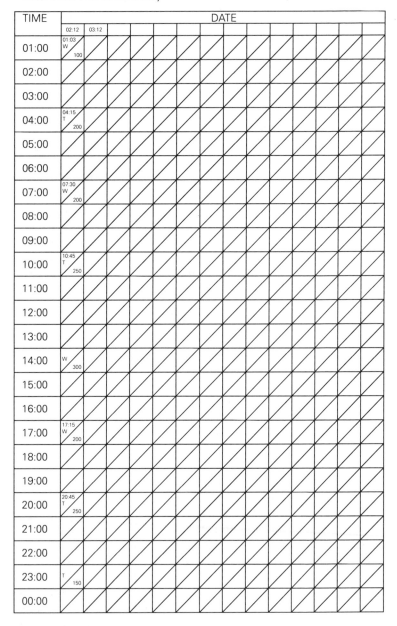

TIME	DATE													
	02:12	03:12												
01:00	01:03 W 100													
02:00														
03:00														
04:00	04:15 T 200													
05:00														
06:00														
07:00	07:30 W 200													
08:00														
09:00														
10:00	10:45 T 250													
11:00														
12:00														
13:00														
14:00	W 300													
15:00														
16:00														
17:00	17:15 W 200													
18:00														
19:00														
20:00	20:45 T 250													
21:00														
22:00														
23:00	T 150													
00:00														

Figure 3.2   Wet/dry/volume chart.

important to record what patients are drinking, particularly if it is alcoholic since this will not only cause increased urine production as the result of osmotic diuresis (see Chapter 4) but may also cause some degree of sedation which would further contribute to the risk of incontinence (see Chapter 7).

Urgency

How much warning a person receives before experiencing an uncontrollable urge to void can be crucial in determining whether he or she is able to maintain continence. There can be few nurses who have not said 'in a minute' to a hospitalized patient who has asked for a bedpan or urinal and returned after the nominal 'minute' to find that the patient has been unable to prevent an episode of incontinence. The length of time a person can 'hold on' for will vary between individuals, but those who have some degree of nervous system deterioration which delays the sensory impulses from the bladder to the micturition control centre, for example many of the elderly, will have delayed awareness of the need to void and will therefore need to have access to toilet facilities more rapidly. The same is true of those who suffer some degree of bladder instability (see Chapter 4) where spurious and powerful sensory impulses are transmitted from the trigone to the spinal cord giving the sensation of an over distended bladder which they find almost impossible to control.

Other factors which need to be considered when addressing the topic of urgency are mobility, manual dexterity and voiding difficulties.

Mobility

It is probably fair to assume that any one of us who is suffering from a degree of reduced mobility will need to exercise more control over bladder emptying than we would if we were fully mobile. It is also true to say that even if someone only has a very short period of time between experiencing an awareness of the need to void and an urgent desire to empty his or her bladder this will present few problems if he or she is positioned close to toilet facilities and is able to reach them quickly. Bearing this in mind it is likely that there are a number of people who have incontinent episodes simply because of their inability to access toilet facilities in time and, although they may well be incontinent by definition, the underlying cause of their incontinence may not be related primarily to a gross dysfunction of their urinary system. This is an area where it is essential not only to carry out a nursing assessment in relation to the person's mobility, but also to ensure that there is physiotherapy involvement so that the cause of this reduced mobility can be identified. This enables the development of a joint plan of care which includes interventions to improve the person's mobility to a level whereby he or she is no longer unable to reach the toilet in time. This is likely to be achieved more easily within an institutional setting where other members of the multidisciplinary team may be more readily available and the care which is given can be more intensive. It is also an area where assessment by an occupational therapist can be extremely useful, particularly if modifications are required to a person's home in order to improve access to, and usability of, the toilet.

Manual dexterity

Individuals' ability to manipulate their clothing can, on occasions, have almost as profound an effect as mobility on the time it takes them to be in a position to void without the risk of having an incontinent episode. People who, for whatever reason, have limited use of their hands or are unable to stand for long enough to take down their underwear, may find that the delay caused by this may be sufficient to lead them to wet their clothing and hence, again by definition, be incontinent in the absence of gross dysfunction. Initial assessment of this again falls to the nursing staff but it is certainly another area where specialist assessment and advice should be sought from the occupational therapist and the physiotherapist.

Voiding difficulties

The most easily noticed, and probably most frequently reported, voiding difficulty is that of pain related to micturition. The most common cause for this is urinary tract infection which normally manifests itself as a burning sensation when passing urine and for a short period afterwards. In more extreme cases it may be described by patients as feeling like passing broken glass or having sandpaper pulled down their urethra and can be very distressing indeed. At times they will also report bladder pain, normally as a dull ache or, if kidney infection is also present, they will complain of pain in the loin area, sometimes unilaterally. Although urinary tract infection does not inevitably lead to incontinence it can produce symptoms of extreme urgency leading to urge incontinence (see Chapter 4). It is important therefore to consider the possibility of urinary tract infection and pay close attention to the colour, turbidity, smell and pH of the urine and perform a dipstick test for all patients who are incontinent (see Appendix A).

The other main area which needs to be assessed in relation to voiding difficulties is whether the patient has any problems with initiating or stopping the stream of urine once he or she has the urge to void since hesitancy and dribbling are not uncommon problems and are relevant when it comes to identifying the cause of incontinence and using appropriate interventions. One cause of hesitancy which should be excluded at this stage is that of embarrassment. It is comparatively common for anybody who has an audience while passing urine to have some difficulty in initiating the flow. This is a particular problem for men due to the design of most lavatories in public places but may also be a problem for women using public lavatories if they feel that someone in the next cubicle will be able to hear them. This is not unduly surprising since we are all brought up not to urinate in public places or in front of other people and may have some difficulty in shedding this conditioned inhibition especially if we are literally rubbing shoulders with strangers who may be discussing the weather, or whistling loudly, in an attempt to cover their own embarrassment at starting to urinate themselves. Although this does not in itself contribute to continence problems, except in very rare cases where individuals are so scared of using a public lavatory that they hold on for an excessive amount of time, it may be identified by someone who is incontinent as yet another problem. If it is perceived as such, then it should be addressed in general terms but it should also be stressed that in reality it has no bearing on the individual's continence problems and as such should cause him or her no further anxiety.

Bowels

Bowel function should be assessed for all people complaining of incontinence regardless of whether it is faecal, urinary or double. It is particularly important in this part of the assessment to exclude constipation, which can not only cause a degree of outflow obstruction but can also contribute to problems of urgency and frequency.

PSYCHOLOGICAL ASSESSMENT

As discussed above, incontinence can carry with it a high level of social stigma (Oliver, 1985; McGrother *et al.*, 1987) and the denial that often accompanies this may make it difficult to gain information from a patient. It is important therefore to gain some idea of the person's attitude to his or her incontinence since an attitude of resignation or apathy towards it will make the task of caring for the individual at best difficult or at worst nigh on impossible, and it may be necessary initially to direct nursing efforts towards developing a positive attitude prior to attempting any interventions directly linked to the incontinence. In extreme cases, where a patient may be suffering from depression related to the incontinence, it would be wise to consider whether an assessment by a psychologist, psychiatric nurse or a trained counsellor would be of more benefit, since it is also possible that the patient's mental state may be causing, or at least be a contributory factor to, the incontinence.

If there is reason to believe that the patient is suffering from an acute or chronic confusional state it may be desirable to perform some type of mental assessment to determine the degree of confusion. This is not strictly necessary, however, for an initial assessment related to the person's incontinence but it is important to determine whether or not he or she is capable of remembering where the toilet facilities are, or of recognizing appropriate places to void. Some patients who are suffering from confusion appear not to be able to recognize overtly the need to void or the fact that they are wet. This means that they are unable to communicate the need to staff or carers. Under these circumstances there may be signs which are unique to the patient that they have a full bladder. There vary from increased restlessness to almost outright aggression and with careful observation it is often possible to recognize that a patient is feeling the need to void prior to his or her becoming wet and take appropriate action to prevent incontinence (see Chapter 7).

ASSESSMENT CHECKLISTS

There are several checklists available for documenting a continence assessment, ranging from the lengthy and highly complex to comparatively simple documents. As long as the main points are included in an assessment the format and length of the documentation matters less than the fact that an assessment has been carried out. A simplified assessment form which is suitable for use in any setting, but particularly where there is no ready access to more in-depth examination facilities (e.g. residential homes or the patient's own home), is shown in Figure 3.3.

If facilities are available for further assessment and examination other categories can be included on the form to cover, for example, invasive urodynamic investigations (see below) and any relevant details which may emerge as the result of a full medical examination (Figure 3.4).

Ideally, the assessment documentation should be used by, and be available to, all staff involved in the patient's care in order to ensure that a comprehensive picture is built up representing the professional opinions of different members of the multidisciplinary team. It is particularly important, however, that any assessment information is signed and dated and that the professional discipline, as well as the name, of the assessor is clearly identifiable.

INVASIVE PROCEDURES AND URODYNAMIC INVESTIGATIONS

As discussed in Chapter 1, there is limited availability of these facilities and it is likely that they will not be available, or necessarily appropriate, to large numbers of the incontinent population. Since the execution and interpretation of the

CONTINENCE ASSESSMENT CHECKLIST

(N.B. This should not be used in isolation, medical assessment and other specialist advice should be sought as appropriate.)

Client Name: .... D.O.B.: .... Date: ....

Dr's Name: .... Assessment carried out by: ....

- When does incontinence occur? (Use wet/dry chart to establish pattern.)

- What signs and symptoms does the client have?
  - Frequency
  - Urgency
  - Leakage on exertion
  - Pain on micturition
  - Difficulty on voiding
  - Dribbling
  - Nocturia
  - Nocturnal enuresis
  - Amount of urine lost
  - Smelly/cloudy urine
  - Passive incontinence

- How long can the client 'hold on'?

- Does the client have any warning?

- Is the client constipated?

- Is the client sufficiently mobile to get to the toilet?

- Can the client manipulate his/her clothing?

---

cont'd

- How does the client feel about the problem?

- Can the client communicate his/her needs?

- Is the client: Fully orientated?
                                     Partially orientated?
                                     Confused?

- Are there problems in the environment which contribute to the client's problems? (Also consider fluid intake and output.)

- Action plan:

Figure 3.3   Basic continence assessment checklist.

majority of these investigations fall within the remit of the medical staff, or nurses working in the field of urodynamics or urology, in-depth discussion of the practicalities of performing them is not appropriate here. It is important, however, to be aware of what the investigations entail and their relevance to the care and management of an incontinent patient in order to be in a position to make appropriate referrals and to give accurate patient education to those who are faced with them.

Residual urine

Measurement of residual urine is probably the most commonly performed invasive procedure related to continence assessment. It is performed by inserting a non-retaining catheter into the bladder after the patient has voided and allowing any urine which is present to drain, removing the catheter and recording the amount collected. The investigation will reveal

CONTINENCE ASSESSMENT CHECKLIST:

Patient Name: D.O.B.:   Date:

Dr's Name: Assessment carried out by:

History of present condition: (including current medications)

Relevant previous history: (including obstetric history)

Physical assessment:
Pattern of incontinence: (see continence chart) Urine/Faeces?
Urinalysis:

Main urinary problems:
Frequency
Urgency
Leakage on exertion
Pain on micturition   at other times
Difficulty in voiding
Dribbling
Nocturia
Nocturnal enuresis

Current strategies used to manage incontinence:
Altered fluid intake
Intermittent self-catheterization   How often?
Indwelling catheter
Forced bladder emptying
Pads   Type   Number used
Penile sheath
Other

Time between sensation of the need to void and incontinence occurring

Bowels:
Constipation/diarrhoea?
Usual pattern
Changes in pattern
Laxatives/anti-diarrhoeals used

General factors:
Mobility   Independent   Aids used
Manual dexterity
Visual problems
Skin condition
Odour
Vaginal/rectal prolapse
Anatomical changes (e.g. atrophy/retraction)
Residual urine
Urodynamic investigations

Social assessment:
Type of housing
Accessibility of toilet
Existing modifications
Level of privacy

cont'd

Washing facilities
Lives alone/with carer
Usual support network
Employment
Social activities
Restrictions resulting from incontinence
Statutory/voluntary service involvement
Laundry facilities

Psychological assessment:
Relationship with carer
Attitude to incontinence
Carer's attitude to incontinence
Level of orientation

General comments:

Action plan:

Figure 3.4 Detailed continence assessment checklist.

whether the patient has a problem emptying his or her bladder completely although residual urine measurements of 5–10 ml are not uncommon and are highly unlikely to be of any significance. As with all invasive bladder procedures there is a risk of introducing infection and the normal precautions which apply to urethral catheterization should be taken (see Chapter 6). Residual urine volumes can also be measured using ultrasound techniques and, although the capital cost of purchasing the equipment may be comparatively high, this method removes the risk of causing direct trauma to the patient and of introducing infection. Equally important is the fact that it also carries less potential for the patient to experience any embarrassment.

Flow rate

The rate at which urine is passed can be measured comparatively simply by use of a modified commode containing a funnel into which the patient voids. The urine is then directed through a flow meter or into a receptacle containing an electronic dipstick which monitors and records the rate of flow in millilitres per second. A reduced flow rate or gross variations in the rate during micturition will yield information with regard to the contractility of the detrusor muscle and the possibility of outflow obstruction. Because of the simplicity of the investigation and its non-invasive nature, it poses few problems for the patient in terms of embarrassment and no risk of trauma or infection.

Cystometrogram

This investigation is used to determine the pressure within the bladder while it is filling. Normally two catheters are inserted into the bladder, one to allow filling of the bladder with normal saline (at room temperature) and the other to measure the pressure in the bladder. A third catheter is inserted into the rectum and serves to measure the intra-abdominal pressure. This is necessary to calculate the true pressure created by the detrusor muscle since any increase in intra-abdominal pressure will cause a rise in bladder pressure which is not attributable to detrusor contractions. The patient is asked to describe the sensation he or she feels during the filling phase and this is then compared with the measured detrusor pressure (i.e. the figure reached by subtracting the intra-abdominal pressure reading obtained from the rectal probe from the reading obtained from the bladder probe). This gives an indication of the detrusor pressure during the filling phase of the bladder. In a further variation of this test, the micturating cystometrogram, the patient is asked to void with the probes still in place thereby giving a reading of the detrusor pressure during the emptying phase. It is normal for the pressure to increase during emptying and then to revert to almost zero. The final stage of this investigation is the removal of the bladder probe which gives an indication of the urethral closing pressure as it is withdrawn from the urethra.

A more complex and potentially more embarrassing addition to the cystometrogram, since it takes place in the x-ray department, is the video cystometrogram which involves the use of a radio-opaque dye (similar to that used for intravenous urograms) which is excreted via the kidneys and hence into the bladder. During this investigation a video recording is taken of the x-ray image of the bladder while it is filling and emptying. By this means, any anatomical abnormalities, such as deformities of the bladder neck, bladder diverticula and new growths of the bladder walls, can be determined.

Cystoscopy

A more direct method of examination is that of cystoscopy. This can be used for direct visualization of the urethra and bladder mucosa and taking biopsies. Under normal circumstances a flexible cystoscope will be used which is inserted under local anaesthetic. The procedure may cause the patient some embarrassment but should not involve any more than slight discomfort.

As mentioned above, invasive procedures may not be necessary for the majority of patients suffering from incontinence. From a nursing viewpoint a full patient assessment and history will be sufficient to obtain the information required to identify a patient's problems and commence appropriate interventions based on a problem solving approach. In broad terms the problems which are likely to be identified are those of frequency, urgency, leakage on exertion, dribbling and difficulty in voiding and lack of awareness of the need to void. These will be considered in detail in the following chapters.

REFERENCES AND FURTHER READING

Brown, P. (1988) Health care and the aged: a nursing perspective, in *Assessment of the Older Person* (ed. P. Brown), Williams and Wilkins, London.

Campbell, J., Finch, D., Allport, C. *et al.* (1985) A theoretical approach to nursing assessment. *Journal of Advanced Nursing*, **10**, 111–15.

Faulkner, A. (1992) *Effective Interaction with Patients*, Churchill Livingstone, Edinburgh.

Hilton, P. and Stanton, S. (1981) Algorithmic method for assessing urinary incontinence in women. *British Medical Journal*, **282**, 940–2.

Kagan, C., Evans, J. and Kay, B. (1986) *A Manual of Interpersonal Skills for Nurses*, Harper and Row, London.

McGrother, C., Castleden, C., Duffin, H. and Clarke, M. (1987) A profile of disordered micturition in the elderly at home. *Age and Ageing*, **16**, 105–10.

Oliver, J. (1985) Fresh and dry? *Nursing Times*, **81**(30), 21.

Roper, N., Logan, W. and Tierney, A. (1990) *The Elements of Nursing: A Model for Nursing Based on a Model of Living*, 3rd edn, Churchill Livingstone, Edinburgh.

4

Frequency and urgency

These two problems are probably those that are most commonly experienced by individuals who may not suffering from any form of incontinence yet are concerned about their urinary function. It is only when a person finds that the urgency is irresistible and there are no toilet facilities available that urge incontinence may result. It is possible to experience a degree of urgency without frequency, as may occur in response to a running tap, immersion in water or when one reaches the toilet after a long period of waiting, when the urge to void is sometimes so great that the individual may pass a very small amount of urine into the urethra. The presence of urine in the urethra further compounds the feeling of urgency and some leakage may occur. Some may consider this to be sufficient cause to label the person incontinent regardless of how infrequently it occurs. This further reinforces the need for a definition such as that in Chapter 1. A degree of measurability when considering incontinence is obviously desirable since there are many people (judging from responses from 'healthy' students and others who have been questioned) who have occasionally experienced such an occurrence but who could not reasonably be classed as incontinent and who certainly do not require any intervention. It is also possible to encounter a situation where there is frequency without urgency – when the desire to void, although occurring at frequent intervals, is not associated with a high level of urgency but is none the less responded to by the individual.

At this point it is important to attempt to reach some objective definition of what constitutes frequency and urgency. The suggestion made in Chapter 3, that voiding any more frequently than 3–6 hourly could be considered as indicative of frequency, is not unreasonable under normal levels of hydration. This means that on average a person will void between three and six times during waking hours in any given 24 hour period with no voiding taking place during sleep (Hilton and Stanton, 1981). This does not however take into account the occasions when hydration levels are above normal and it is not uncommon for an individual who has been drinking large amounts of fluid to void a 'normal' amount of urine (i.e. 300–400 ml) twice or even three times an hour. The effect of fluid intake can only really be determined by the use of a comprehensive assessment of intake and output as described in Chapter 3. It is probably fair to say therefore that anyone who passes small amounts of urine (less than 200 ml) more often than once every three hours is suffering from frequency. If an individual is passing large amounts of urine, in the absence of an abnormally large intake, at frequent intervals it may be indicative of some underlying disorder such as diabetes mellitus or diabetes insipidus both of which can lead to polyuria (normally in excess of 3 litres per day). Further investigations should be carried out by the medical staff to identify the cause.

COMMON CAUSES OF FREQUENCY AND URGENCY AND RELATED PHYSIOLOGY

Diuretic therapy

The majority of patients undergoing diuretic therapy will produce more urine in a shorter period of time than is customary for them. This can result in both frequency and urgency leading in some cases to urge incontinence. The exception to this is when the patient is severely oliguric or even anuric (as in the case of acute cardiac failure) when even the use of diuretics may have little effect on urine production. The amount of urine produced and the speed at which it is produced is dependent to a large extent on the type of diuretic used and the route of administration (Trounce and Gould, 1990).

Loop diuretics   This group of diuretics affects the reabsorption of water from the loop of Henle and is also known as 'high ceiling' diuretics. The onset of action is particularly rapid, often within 20 minutes of administration. Large quantities of urine are produced within a short period of time, normally 2–3 hours. Of the diuretics in common use, this group is the most likely to precipitate urge incontinence.

Thiazide diuretics   These produce a less powerful effect than the loop diuretics and are therefore less likely to cause continence problems. They act on the tubules of the kidney and the diuresis which they produce is slower in onset and longer in duration.

The degree to which a person will be able to compensate for the increased urine production will be dependent upon a number of factors such as bladder capacity, nervous system controls and the availability of toilet facilities. If the episodes of incontinence coincide with the administration of the diuretic therapy then this suggests very strongly that the medication is the causative factor and there are then various interventions which should be considered. Firstly it is important to liaise with the doctor responsible for prescribing the diuretic in the first place. It is possible that the doctor may review the need for using a diuretic at all, reduce the dosage, alter the timing of administration or change the prescription to a slower acting drug which will not produce such a dramatic diuresis but which will still be effective. In some circumstances this may be sufficient to prevent the incontinence from occurring but, if none of the above are feasible or if they do not improve the situation, then other interventions should be used. The most important aspect to note is how soon incontinence occurs after administration of the drug. Once this is determined appropriate toilet facilities can be made available at this time and for the period during which the action of the drug is still causing difficulties for the patient. Initially this will involve careful observation and timing, but in this case a pattern should be easily identifiable and the incidence of incontinent episodes will be reduced significantly.

Anxiety

This is probably the most common reason for a person to experience frequency of micturition, often without urgency. In the absence of any bladder or sphincter dysfunction this should not in itself be a reason for incontinence occurring, it does, however, aggravate any underlying disorder and can cause a degree of stress if not explained to the patient. The reasons for frequency when a person is anxious may be twofold. Firstly there is a psychological element which may be most apparent if the person is going to have difficulty in going to the toilet for a period of time (e.g. during an examination). This can lead to an individual making several visits to the toilet where he or she will only pass a few millilitres of urine prior to the stressful event which is anticipated. This should not cause a long term problem unless the individual is regularly exposed to such events when the pattern of frequent voiding can become a habit. The second element relates to the nervous control of micturition. When exposed to stress the 'fight or flight' reaction comes into effect which involves, amongst other things, increased activity of the sympathetic nervous system (Tortora and Anagnostakos, 1990). This leads to an enhanced awareness of the sensory impulses from the bladder trigone and a subsequent feeling of urgency to void regardless of the amount of urine in the bladder. Again this should not in itself lead to incontinence but can be disturbing if it occurs on a regular basis and the potential is there for both these elements to aggravate an underlying problem or in extreme cases lead to incontinent episodes. In neither case should incontinence be a problem when the person is asleep since there will be no awareness of the anxiety-producing stimulus.

Little can be done, other than offering reassurance and explanation, for occasional frequency resulting from stress related causes. Frequency can become a habit, however, for some people who become used to voiding at the first sensation of bladder fullness. Under such circumstances it may be necessary to initiate a programme of bladder training, as would be done for detrusor instability (see below).

CAUSES OF IRRITATION TO THE BLADDER AND URETHRA

Any irritation of the bladder or urethral mucosa can lead to frequency and urgency. In the case of the bladder the irritation leads to abnormal stimulation of the trigone which in turn results in spurious sensory impulses being sent to the spinal cord and brain. The causes of irritation, broadly divided, are discussed as follows.

Urinary tract infection

Infection of any part of the urinary tract can lead to inflamation of the bladder lining and trigonal stimulation. In the case of glomerulonephritis or pyelonephritis, stimulation of the trigone may be minimal (particularly if the person is drinking large amounts of fluid which serves to flush out the infective agent). Under these circumstances the person is likely to complain of pyrexia and loin pain in association with any urinary symptoms which are reported. These symptoms may be absent in the case of patients with chronic bacteriuria who remain asymptomatic for indefinite periods of time and may only experience problems if the infection becomes acute. When urinary tract infection is present it may be sufficient in itself to cause urge incontinence or it may serve to aggravate other bladder problems. It should always be excluded as a contributory factor since persistent infection is not only a risk to the patient but will also hinder any attempts to regain continence. Often visual examination of the urine coupled with a dipstick test for nitrate will be sufficient to indicate clearly that infection is present, but it is desirable to ensure that a specimen is sent for culture and sensitivity to identify the causative organism and appropriate treatment.

Minor trauma to the urethra

Urethral trauma may be caused by a direct blow to the urethra, by energetic sexual intercourse, masturbation or the insertion of foreign bodies into the urethra. The result of this is damage to the urethral mucosa which becomes inflamed and irritated leading to pain and a sensation of urgency. This is further aggravated by the presence of urine since the underlying cells of the urethra are no longer fully protected by the mucosa. Although the condition is uncomfortable and there is potential for infection at the site of the damage it will normally resolve itself within a few days if the urethra is treated gently and is not exposed to further damage. Raising the pH of the urine may also help to relieve the discomfort, and hence the urgency. This can be achieved by taking proprietary preparations such as potassium citrate which are available without prescription, although patients should be advised that if the symptoms persist for more than three days with no resolution they should seek further advice.

Chemical irritation

Even in the absence of urethral trauma irritation can be caused by changes in the chemical composition of the urine. The most common cause of this is a low urinary pH (see Appendix A) which not only irritates the urethra but also the bladder mucosa itself. This can be responsible for the problems encountered in non-infective cystitis and again should respond well to lowering the pH of the urine.

Another factor to be considered in relation to the chemical composition of the urine is its concentration. Many people who suffer from incontinence are tempted to restrict their fluid intake in order to reduce the amount of urine produced. This does occur, but the inevitable consequence is more concentrated urine which may serve to exacerbate any underlying problems of detrusor instability or even cause sufficient irritation in its own right to lead to frequency and urgency. In some cases reduced fluid intake may be as a result of decreased thirst sensation or an inability to drink independently. Loss of independence with regard to fluid intake may occur for a number of reasons ranging from dysphagia to an inability to reach or hold a glass or cup. In both these cases it is clearly the responsibility of the carers to ensure that the person's fluid intake is monitored and that sufficient fluid is consumed. In an institutional setting where professional care staff are involved this should present fewer difficulties than a community setting, but even here the problem can be minimized by ensuring that both patients themselves and their carers are informed of the importance of maintaining an adequate fluid intake. Fluid restriction is not, therefore, a suitable means of controlling incontinence. The timing of fluid intake, however, can be manipulated and may prove useful particularly if someone has problems with nocturia or nocturnal enuresis. Under these circumstances it may be helpful to ensure that all or the majority of a person's intake takes place before a set time in the evening. This allows for the bulk of urine production to take place prior to the person going to bed and a decrease in urine production during the night with a consequent decrease in the risk of incontinent episodes. What must be emphasized, however, is that over a 24 hour period the total fluid intake should remain within the normal range of 1500–2500 ml. This technique may also be useful before a journey or outing where toilet facilities may not be readily available.

A further source of chemical irritation is direct contact of the urethral mucosa with an irritant such as soap, or occasionally toilet cleaner or bleach in the case of men sitting down to use the toilet, which may cause itching or pain in the distal section of the urethra. Although there is no direct bladder involvement this will lead to frequency which, unless the irritant has caused damage to the urethra, should resolve rapidly once the chemical is washed out of the urethra.

Bladder stones

These may originate in the bladder itself or arise as the result of a small stone being passed from the kidney into the bladder. It is unusual for a stone to form in the bladder without some focus for its growth such as a residual fragment of encrustation from a catheter which has been removed (Blandy, 1989). Under normal circumstances stones originating from the kidney would be passed through the urethra on micturition and the presence of these in the bladder is often associated with a degree of outflow obstruction which prevents this from happening.

Any foreign body which is present in the bladder will not only cause direct stimulation of the trigone when it comes in contact with it but may also cause trauma to the urothelium resulting in further inflamation and irritation, both of which will lead to frequency. Coupled with this patients may complain of pain, often worse on standing or walking when the stone is in direct contact with the trigone, and haematuria may also be detectable. Removal of stones is normally done via the urethra unless they are particularly large when open surgery may be required.

New growths of the bladder

Whether benign or malignant any growth on the bladder mucosa may cause inflammation and irritation of the trigone.

In extreme circumstances the size of the growth itself may reduce functional bladder capacity to such a degree that frequency is inevitable. Coupled with this the patient may complain of haematuria, a characteristic sign of bladder cancer, some dysuria and other signs which are associated with metastatic spread of the tumour. The definitive diagnosis of this is dependent primarily on cystoscopy and biopsy of the lesion and any patient with persistent haematuria in the absence of any other known cause should be referred to a doctor as soon as possible.

Detrusor instability

Although all of the above can be responsible for episodic urge incontinence the commonest cause of persistent frequency and urgency leading to incontinence is detrusor instability or unstable bladder. This is sometimes referred to as neurogenic bladder, but this term has the potential to be misleading since it can cover a variety of conditions relating to disruption of the nervous control of micturition and it is not therefore a particularly helpful one to use. Detrusor instability results in powerful sensory impulses being transmitted from the trigone to the spinal cord during the filling phase of the bladder. These may occur when there is as little as 30 ml of urine in the bladder and, as in the case of irritation to the trigone, the sensation is perceived by the patient as having a full bladder which he or she needs to empty immediately. This sensation is usually coupled with strong detrusor contractions which in turn lead to urge incontinence since the individual is unable to exercise sufficient inhibitory control to prevent them taking place. The cause of detrusor instability is often undetermined although it can be associated with underlying nervous system disorders such as multiple sclerosis.

Detrusor instability leads to a particularly disabling form of incontinence since the need to void with such frequency may lead individuals to limit their lifestyle to such an extent that they are not prepared to leave their homes and are therefore unable to perform their normal activities of living. Any infection or other source of irritation to the bladder mucosa will further aggravate the condition and may, in some cases, be the precipitating factor which leads the patient to seek help. The nursing interventions related to unstable bladder hinge on a programme of bladder training. (This should not be confused with toilet training which is a completely different process used when teaching a child to acquire continence skills.)

BLADDER TRAINING

The key to successful bladder training is motivation both on the part of the patient and the nurse (Holmes, 1990; Kennedy, 1992). It may be a comparatively long process taking some weeks and there are likely to be times during this period when the patient becomes disillusioned as the result of 'failures' and 'accidents'. Support from the nurse and others involved with patients in their home setting is of paramount importance at this time. A baseline chart will have been maintained to record when incontinence occurs and when the patient uses the toilet successfully. The first stage of the process is to maintain an accurate record of how long he or she can hold on for between the onset of the sensation to void and bladder emptying taking place. This may require the use of a stopwatch since this time interval may only be a matter of seconds for some patients and is frequently less than a minute. Once this has been established the patient is asked to attempt to hold on either for specified time periods, which may be as little as a minute longer than normally achieved, or if this proves to be difficult to hold on for as long as he or she is able and record this time. This is perhaps the most difficult part of the process since patients are likely to have attempted this themselves at some stage and may well be convinced that it is an impossibility. Under these circumstances it is up to the nurse to provide a high level of support and encouragement. Straightforward explanations to the patient must emphasize that, although it will be very difficult at first, it is in reality a very similar process to that which the patient probably carried out prior to experiencing problems of urgency when he or she needed to void and could not find a toilet. Reassurance that improvement can be quite rapid will also help and if the training programme is working this will be reinforced by the stopwatch record which should indicate gradually increasing time intervals. It must be remembered that, for individuals who have been used to having to void immediately they feel the urge, any increase in this time interval, howevŕ small, can be seen as a measure of success.

Once a degree of control has been achieved, and the patient's level of confidence has increased, it is usually possible to begin to set longer time intervals for the patient to aim for between voiding. Again these need to be extended gradually and each time interval should be maintained for approximately one week. It should be emphasized to the patient that the toilet can be used between these times if it is absolutely necessary and that this should not be viewed as a failure. The patient should simply record the times when it was required. If it is apparent that the time interval which was agreed initially is too long then this should be re-negotiated to a more realistic interval which can then be increased as the patient feels able. If the urgency is not too severe it may be possible to omit the first part of the process and proceed directly to set time intervals and the feasibility of this should be assessed for each individual. The use of pads as a safeguard during the training programme may help to increase the patient's sense of security and this will need to be discussed with him or her. An over reliance on pads may lead to decreased levels of motivation, however. If this is suspected it should be discussed with the patient and an agreement reached as to how long he or she will continue to use them.

Overall the whole programme may take as little as eight weeks to complete but it must be pointed out to the patient that it is not possible to predict the exact length of time since there can be wide variations between individuals in the rate of improvement. The use of pelvic floor exercise during the training programme may also be advisable and will help to reduce the incidence of leakage.

Drug therapy for detrusor instability

This is one of the few occasions when the use of drugs for incontinence can cause a dramatic improvement in the condition. Often drug therapy on its own can be sufficient to relieve all the symptoms of frequency and urgency or alternatively it can be used in conjunction with a bladder training programme. The principle behind the drug therapy relies on the fact that the sensory impulses from the bladder are carried by the sympathetic nervous system and that any drug which has an anticholinergic effect will serve to dampen down the impulses to an acceptable level which enables the patient to exercise sufficient control to avoid incontinence (Trounce and Gould, 1990). It is important to provide the patient with information about the side effects of the drug therapy since in some cases they may be sufficient to cause lack of compliance with the treatment. The likelihood of this happening will be reduced if the patient is warned that they may occur and reassured that it is not abnormal. Since the drugs have an effect on the sensory impulses there is a risk that retention of urine may occur if the dose is too large and it is particularly important to warn the patient of this. Informed patients can take prompt action and seek assistance if such effects occur. Good information giving also reduces the risk of the patient taking more than the prescribed dose in an attempt to speed up or initiate an improvement in his or her condition.

Patients who have severe problems as a result of their frequency and urgency may require surgical intervention, although this can be seen as a last resort and will not be necessary in the vast majority of cases.

REFERENCES AND FURTHER READING

Blandy, J. (1989) *Lecture Notes on Urology*, 4th edn, Blackwell Scientific Publications, Oxford.

Hilton, P. and Stanton, S. (1981) Algorithmic method for assessing urinary incontinence in elderly women. *British Medical Journal*, 282, 940–2.

Holmes, P. (1990) Mind over bladder. *Nursing Times*, **86**(4), 16–17.

Kennedy, A. (1992) Bladder re-education for the promotion of continence, in *Clinical Nursing Practice* (ed B. Roe), Prentice Hall, New York.

Tortora, G. and Anagnostakos, N. (1990) *Principles of Anatomy and Physiology*, 6th edn, Harper and Row, London. Chapter 26.

Trounce, J. and Gould, D. (1990) *Clinical Pharmacology for Nurses*, 13th edn, Churchill Livingstone, Edinburgh.

5

Leakage on exertion

This problem is commonly referred to as 'stress incontinence'.
This term does have its drawbacks, however, not least that the
stress which is referred to has no connection whatsoever with
emotional stress. It refers solely to a rise in intra-abdominal
pressure which results from some form of physical stress or
exertion. This confusion is not restricted to members of the
general public and it is not uncommon for both qualified and
student nurses to associate the term with anxiety-provoking
events.

It is important to remember exactly what constitutes leakage
of urine. According to the definition proposed in Chapter 1,
any amount of urine that is lost can be considered to be leakage
and if it happens twice or more a month the person can be
considered to be incontinent (Thomas *et al.*, 1980). This needs
to be emphasized at this point because the leakage which
occurs with exertion can range from a few drops of urine which
are barely noticeable to a bladderful. In the former case it is not
uncommon for an individual to minimize the loss to such an
extent that it is also ignored by nursing staff and consequently
no advice is given and no action taken to remedy the problem.
The level of exertion which is required to cause leakage also
varies between individuals. This too is important to consider
since a person who only experiences leakage on major exertion,
such as running or other sporting activities, is likely to express
less concern about it than someone who experiences leakage
on laughing or coughing. In reality any person who experiences
any degree of leakage, even if it only occurs as a result of gross
physical activity, should be offered advice and support by
nursing staff since the likelihood is that, untreated, the problem
will get worse as the person gets older and early intervention

can not only solve the immediate problem but also prevent it recurring or worsening.

CAUSES OF LEAKAGE

One reason why there may be considerable differences in the amount of urine lost on exertion is that various factors may be involved in the cause of the leakage. In some cases a cough or sneeze may be responsible for stimulating an already unstable bladder to contract (i.e. it is the instability which is the true cause of the incontinence as opposed to the exertion) and this may be the problem which the patient presents with. Careful assessment and the use of urodynamic investigations will confirm whether or not this is the underlying cause and appropriate interventions should be instigated (Chapter 4). Equally individuals with atonic bladder (see Chapter 6) are likely to experience more leakage and dribbling when exerting themselves – although this situation may be more easily recognized without the use of urodynamic investigations since leakage will occur even without exertion.

Both of the above situations may be described in broad terms as 'stress incontinence', but it is important to distinguish between the above which are related to bladder dysfunction, and what is described as 'genuine' stress incontinence which strictly speaking is associated with an incompetent sphincter mechanism.

ANATOMY AND PHYSIOLOGY RELATED
TO LEAKAGE ON EXERTION

In all cases of leakage, regardless of the underlying cause, the common factor is a rise in intra-abdominal pressure which in turn increases the pressure exerted on the bladder itself. As previously suggested intra-abdominal pressure may rise as the result of a number of different activities. Commonly these are as follows:

- sneezing
- coughing
- laughing
- physical exercise
- breathing in deeply

- standing up from sitting
- sexual intercourse.

In all of these cases the pressure is transferred to the bladder as a result of direct contraction of the abdominal muscles, pressure from the diaphragm and abdominal contents or direct external pressure.

In the case of an underlying bladder instability, the rise in intra-abdominal pressure results in a sufficient rise in the internal bladder pressure to stimulate the trigone to transmit sensory impulses to the spinal cord with the result that the person experiences urgency to void and is likely to empty the bladder contents completely. Coupled with leakage on exertion, such an individual is also likely to experience urgency, and probably frequency, at other times not associated with exertion. This should be investigated at the assessment stage, since the persons who are not experiencing leakage at any other time may fail to mention that they have other urinary problems because the times when they are wet are the most significant to them. If an underlying instability is suspected a combination of pelvic floor exercises and bladder training (as described in Chapter 4) should be instituted.

In the case of an individual with an atonic bladder it is likely that leakage will occur in the absence of exertion but be more pronounced when the intra-abdominal pressure is increased. If this is suspected then assessment and interventions for atonic bladder should be carried out as described in Chapter 6.

The final case is that of leakage on exertion due to an incompetent sphincter or so called 'genuine' stress incontinence. This term is itself open to a degree of misinterpretation since some authors (Bates *et al.*, 1975) would define this as the leakage of urine in the absence of detrusor activity. If this definition is to be accepted then leakage on exertion as a result of atonic bladder could also be considered to be genuine stress incontinence since there is an absence of detrusor contraction although the interventions required differ greatly from those which would be employed to treat leakage due to an incompetent sphincter. Since detrusor instability and atonic bladder are addressed elsewhere, the remainder of this chapter will concern itself solely with leakage as a result of an incompetent sphincter mechanism and any future reference to stress incontinence can be taken to refer to this.

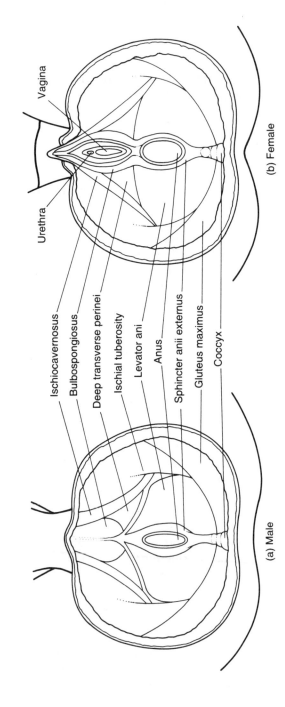

Figure 5.1 Pelvic floor musculature.

Vagina

Urethra

Ischiocavernosus

Bulbospongiosus

Deep transverse perinei

Ischial tuberosity

Levator ani

Anus

Sphincter anii externus

Gluteus maximus

Coccyx

(a) Male

(b) Female

The closure mechanism that can be considered to be of most importance in stress incontinence is that provided by the pelvic floor muscles. In broad terms the pelvic floor can be seen to consist of a group of muscles, the levator ani which divides to form the pubococcygeus and the ileococcygeus, and the coccygeus muscle itself. These form a hammock like structure which serves to support the contents of the abdominal cavity (Figure 5.1).

The urethra, rectum and, in women, the vagina all pass through the muscle network and, because of the close association of these muscles with the muscles of the abdomen, any contraction of the abdominal muscles is transferred to the pelvic floor which contracts almost simultaneously to increase the pressure exerted on the urethra and the rectum to prevent leakage of urine or faeces. Coupled with this ability to respond rapidly to a rise in intra-abdominal pressure the pelvic floor muscles also provide a longer term function of support contributing to the maintenance of continence.

Stress incontinence results predominantly from some form of weakness or damage to these muscles which may result in either a weakness of the sphincter itself or an inability of the muscles to function adequately due to anatomical changes in the position of the bladder or of the uterus. The group who are predominantly affected by stress incontinence are women and although it is a problem which is almost exclusive to females (Norton, 1986) it can occur in men usually following prostatectomy and they should not be ignored as a group who may benefit from pelvic floor assessment and treatment.

Various factors are responsible for this gender determined distribution, the main one being pregnancy and childbirth. In pregnancy there is an increased pressure on the pelvic floor musculature as a result of the weight of the foetus and the amniotic fluid within the uterus. This may in itself be responsible for sufficient stretching of the muscles whilst the woman is pregnant to cause a temporary stress incontinence which resolves once she has given birth. This abnormal strain on the muscles may, however, cause sufficient damage to leave the woman with a residual weakness which persists even when the pressure is removed. Another factor which serves to aggravate this situation is the process of vaginal birth itself. During delivery the pelvic floor muscles are further stressed and

stretched which, even if the woman has experienced no difficulties during the pregnancy, may be sufficient to cause her
to suffer from stress incontinence afterwards (Sleep and Grant,
1987; Jonasson, Larsson and Pschera, 1989).

Another significant factor with regard to stress incontinence
is obesity. Although the exact definition of obesity may vary
somewhat, depending on which height/weight chart is being
used, any excess weight which is being carried can lead to a
degree of stress incontinence. This is particularly significant if
an individual already has a weakened pelvic floor and any
extra pressure on the muscles, even that resulting from mild
weight gain, may be sufficient to cause incontinence. The
mechanism of this is again related simply to strain on the
muscles caused by excess weight in the abdominal cavity.

In both of the above cases the onset of incontinence may be
very rapid or it may be delayed for several years and the
problem may not manifest itself until the person is elderly.
This is associated with the fact that (as discussed in Chapter 1)
part of the normal ageing process is loss of muscle tone and
elasticity. If the pelvic floor muscles are undamaged and fully
functional prior to this there should not be a significant problem. If however they have been subjected to long term stress
and no action has been taken to counteract this any further
weakness will serve to compound the underlying problem and
may precipitate the onset of incontinence.

Any changes which affect the normal anatomical relationship
of the urethra to the pelvic floor such as prolapse of the uterus,
rectum or in some cases the bladder neck may also result in
stress incontinence. In all of these circumstances the patient is
likely to need some form of corrective surgery to restore the
gross anatomy to normal before any nursing interventions to
promote continence can be undertaken. As such these conditions fall outside the remit of this book although following
surgery the nurse again has a role to play in educating and
supporting the patient with regard to retraining of the pelvic
floor.

RETRAINING OF THE PELVIC FLOOR MUSCLES

The first stage of any programme designed to exercise the
pelvic floor muscles is identification of which muscles are

actually involved in the process. Although this may appear to be comparatively straightforward a number of people seem to have great difficulty with this and as a result either perform pelvic floor exercise ineffectually or give up on them altogether. Perhaps the simplest way to identify the muscles initially is to ask the person to attempt to stop urinating in mid-void. Someone who is capable of doing this is likely to be able to recognize which muscle groups are being used and the associated sensations and continue to use them at other times. For some individuals this is not possible either due to a severely weakened pelvic floor or a general inability to control specific muscle groups which prevents them from stopping the flow of urine. Although stopping mid-flow is a useful technique for muscle identification, and has some practical application in terms of being able to control micturition once started, should the need arise, it does have the potential to lead to a sudden rise in detrusor pressure with the associated risk of ureteric reflux and renal damage. It may also cause particular problems for individuals who suffer from recurrent infective cystitis. In women the effectiveness of the pelvic floor contraction can be assessed by the nurse or by the patient themselves by insertion of one or two fingers into the lower part of the vagina. The woman is then instructed to contract her vagina and the degree of 'squeeze' noted. A more accurate and objective measure of the effectiveness of pelvic floor contraction is the use of a perineometer. This is a device which consists of a

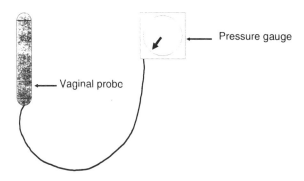

Figure 5.2 Perineometer.

pressure sensitive probe which is inserted into the vagina and attached to a gauge which can be read by the patient or the nurse (Figure 5.2). This may be used purely for assessment purposes or as an aid to any exercise regime which has been instituted.

In men pelvic floor function can be assessed by the insertion of a gloved and lubricated finger into the rectum and again any increase in pressure is noted when the patient is instructed to squeeze. If a man is reluctant to have this assessment performed even after the importance of it has been explained to him some evaluation of the pelvic floor function can be obtained by pressing two fingers onto the mid-line of the perineum behind the scrotum which can be felt to rise slightly if the muscles are functional.

STARTING AN EXERCISE PROGRAMME

Once it has been established that an individual can identify and use the correct muscles in isolation an exercise programme can be negotiated. One of the most important elements to emphasize at the outset is that increasing pelvic floor tone, particularly if the weakness is long standing, can take several months. A high level of perseverance in carrying out the exercises will be required if they are to be successful. Because of this it is essential to check that any instructions which are given to patients are fully understood by them and also that they are reinforced by written information. An individualized plan of exercise should be drawn up with each patient which is reviewed at regular intervals. This not only provides the opportunity to give ongoing support and encouragement but also to monitor any progress. This will help to increase the patient's motivation to carry out the exercises. Individuals should also be encouraged to keep a record of any incontinent episodes and whether or not they have have actually carried out the exercises.

Two forms of pelvic floor exercise are commonly recommended. The first of these is designed to increase the tone of the slow twitch muscle fibres of the external sphincter. The patient is instructed to carry out the exercise on an hourly basis as follows:

1. Sitting or standing contract the pelvic floor muscles and hold for a count of five seconds.
2. Relax the muscles completely for five seconds.
3. Repeat steps 1 and 2 up to a maximum of 10 times.
4. Carry out this cycle five times resting for one minute between each cycle.

The above is of course a very broad generalization and some patients may not be able to hold their contraction for as long as five seconds while some may be able to hold it for longer. In the former situation there is likely to be rapid demotivation on the part of the patients since they may consider that they have failed in the very early stages of the programme, and in the latter the muscles are not truly being exercised since they are not having to exert any effort to maintain the contraction. What is important is that the exercises are carried out on an hourly basis if possible and that the time which an individual can hold the contraction for is assessed, a realistic goal set and the exercise programme evaluated and reviewed accordingly. In this way it should be possible gradually to increase the length of time for which the contraction can be held and obtain maximum benefit from the exercises.

The second form of exercise is aimed at improving the function of the rapid twitch muscles which are active in response to a rise in intra-abbdominal pressure. In this the patient is instructed to perform five to 10 (the exact number again needs to be negotiated with the patient) rapid contractions and relaxations of the pelvic floor. This can be performed either in isolation from the first exercise or immediately following it but need not be performed as frequently as the slow twitch exercises.

Pads may be used initially but an over reliance on their use should be discouraged once there is some improvement in the control which the person is able to exercise. As an added safeguard patients can be advised to ensure that they perform a conscious contraction of the muscles prior to undertaking any activity that may cause leakage and attempt to keep them contracted until the activity is completed. This should not be confused with carrying out a full exercise programme prior to activity since this has the potential to result in muscle fatigue and hence a reduced efficiency.

An exercise regime such as that described above does of course require full co-operation from the patient and would be impossible to institute with any patient suffering from a confusional state. Under these circumstances some improvement in pelvic floor function may be obtained by increasing exercise generally or by the use of specific exercises which although not utilising the pelvic floor muscles in isolation will involve them albeit peripherally (Gordon and Logue, 1985). One means of doing this is to place a pillow or cushion between the patient's knees and ask him or her to grip it. The nurse then kneels in front of the patient and holds the pillow and gently rocks backwards and forwards. This movement helps to stimulate rythmic contractions of the muscles of the thighs and also the pelvic floor (Figure 5.3).

The practicality of performing this form of exercise on a

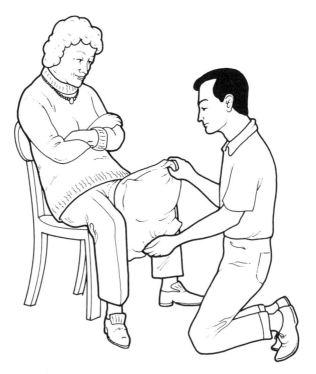

Figure 5.3 Position for performing 'passive' pelvic floor exercises.

regular basis is doubtful as is its overall efficacy, however any form of exercise is probably preferable to none.

The problem of excess weight should also be addressed during the exercise programme and if necessary the dietician should be involved in this, particularly if the patient has experienced difficulty with weight loss. This is an important element of the programme since, as mentioned previously, any weight gain will serve to aggravate the problem if the pelvic floor is already weakened and losing weight may in itself result in a significant reduction in the number of episodes of leakage and, in some cases, solve the problem altogether.

Once continence has been regained the frequency of pelvic floor exercises can be reduced to once or twice per day in order to maintain the muscle tone which has been developed but they should not be stopped altogether, a fact which should be impressed on the patient.

AIDS TO PELVIC FLOOR TRAINING

The perineometer

As previously mentioned a perineometer can be used to measure the strength of pelvic floor contractions and provide an objective reading. The use of this in the longer term following assessment may be helpful to provide the patient with visual feedback as to the progress being made and thus increase motivation levels. The other advantage of this is that target pressures can be set for the patient to aim for which can be included in their plan of care. If however no improvement is evident this may have the opposite effect and demotivate the patient completely. It may be advantageous to consider the use of a perineometer only if the individual appears to be losing interest in performing the exercises with no added incentive.

Vaginal cones

The use of vaginal cones in pelvic floor training has been growing in popularity since they were first introduced by Plevnik in 1985 (Plevnik, 1985; Peattie and Plevnik, 1988). They usually consist of a set of three, or five, differentially weighted cones and their use almost constitutes a form of vaginal weight

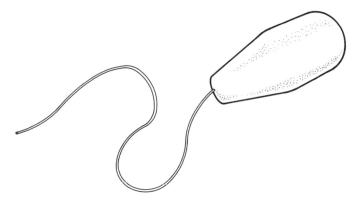

Figure 5.4 Vaginal cones.

training. The aim of the programme is to start with the cone of lowest weight and gradually work up through the weights to heavier cones (Figure 5.4).

Although the manufacturers' instructions for their use differ slightly the general principle is that the patient should start the programme by inserting the lightest cone into the vagina and attempting to hold it there for a period of about 15 minutes once or twice a day for an unspecified number of days while standing up or walking around. If the cone slips out of the vagina during this period it should be re-inserted as many times as is necessary and the exercise continued. After 15 minutes the cone should be removed, washed with soap and water, dried and stored in the container provided. Once the individual is capable of retaining the lightest cone she then progresses to the next heaviest and repeats the same procedure. It should be emphasized to the patient that, like pelvic floor exercise themselves, this method may take several weeks to improve the muscle tone and that not all patients are capable of retaining the heavier cones.

An alternative to the use of vaginal cones which serves to stimulate and exercise the fast twitch muscle fibres is the insertion of a Foley catheter into the vagina which is then inflated with air or water (Laycock, 1987). This is then withdrawn by the patient who is instructed to attempt to grip the balloon in the vagina during withdrawal. This method is more restrictive than using cones since it is more limiting in terms of the activities which patients can perform whilst carrying out the exercise and requires a period of time (usually about 10 minutes) set aside specifically for this purpose. Neither of these methods is recommended during menstuation and they should not be used if there is any suspicion of vaginal infection. If infection does occur during the programme it should be investigated and treated accordingly and an effort made to ascertain the cause since it could be related, amongst other things, to inadequate cleaning and storage of the cones or catheter.

Electrical stimulation

Although the use of electrotherapy has traditionally been the domain of physiotherapists there is no reason why, with appropriate training, nurses should not become more involved in this field. The principle behind electrotherapy is that muscle fibres are stimulated to contract when exposed to a controlled electric current. This in effect allows passive exercise of the pelvic floor to be carried out. There are various forms of electrotherapy available which, although differing in their detailed application, all rely on similar principles to achieve an improvement in the patient's condition.

Both of the above, in isolation, may be capable of improving the problem of stress incontinence without the use of traditional pelvic floor exercise but ideally they should be combined with a regular exercise programme, not only because this is likely to increase the speed of improvement but also to decrease the likelihood of the patient developing an over reliance on external aids.

AIDS FOR THE MANAGEMENT OF STRESS INCONTINENCE

Various aids are available to manage stress incontinence that can be used to prevent leakage either whilst the patient is carrying out an exercise programme or, more appropriately, if all attempts to re-train the pelvic floor have failed. All of the aids available rely on pressure being exerted on the urethra via the anterior vaginal wall.

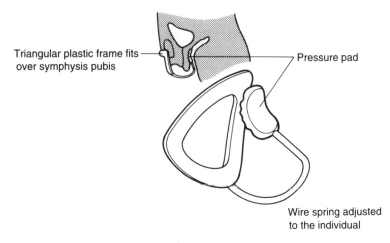

Triangular plastic frame fits over symphysis pubis

Pressure pad

Wire spring adjusted to the individual

Figure 5.5 Edwards device.

The Edwards device

This consists of a shaped metal spring (Figure 5.5) one end of which is inserted into the vagina whilst the other end is lodged over the symphysis pubis. The size and tension of the spring can be adjusted to suit the individual patient. Nevertheless, there is still some risk of pressure necrosis occurring in the vagina, so this device should only be used under close supervision by the person responsible for supplying and fitting it. The spring must be removed for micturition to take place.

Ring pessaries

These may either be indwelling or removable. The indwelling ring pessary is normally inserted by a gynaecologist and sits in the upper part of the vagina just under the cervix. They are comparatively rigid devices and are commonly used if there is evidence of vaginal prolapse. Their function is to support the prolapse whilst at the same time exerting a small amount of pressure on the anterior vaginal wall thus reducing the incidence of leakage. Once inserted they can remain *in situ* for a period of months following which the pessary is removed, the vaginal walls examined and a new pessary inserted. The main complication of using this form of management is the potential for pressure necrosis of the cervix or vaginal wall.

Removable pessaries, which are inserted by patients themselves following instruction, sit in the same position as the ring pessary. One type consists of a soft silicone ring which has a balloon on one of its surfaces. The balloon is positioned anteriorly and is inflated using a syringe via the inflation channel, the valve of which remains outside the vagina. When the woman wishes to pass urine the balloon is deflated and following micturition the position of the pessary is checked and the balloon re-inflated. This device again has the potential to produce pressure necrosis and should be removed at night.

Tampons

Large tampons designed for the absorption of menstrual fluid may provide sufficient pressure on the urethra to reduce or prevent leakage. They do, however, have the disadvantage that they can cause dryness and soreness in the vagina particularly if they are used for long periods of time in the absence of menstrual fluid. If this method of control does prove to be suitable it may be more appropriate for the woman to use a foam tampon specifically designed for this purpose which, because of its reduced absorbency, is less likely to create a problem with soreness whilst still maintaining sufficient pressure to prevent leakage.

LEAKAGE DURING SEXUAL INTERCOURSE

Although leakage during intercourse may be associated with unstable bladder and bladder spasm it can also occur as a result of the physical exertion associated with sexual activity. This can be a particularly embarrassing problem for both men and women and must be handled with great sensitivity by the nurse. The most effective management for this in the short term is for the individual to empty the bladder as completely as possible prior to intercourse taking place which will greatly reduce the risk of leakage and the amount of urine lost. Coupled with this the position in which intercourse takes place can be altered (if both partners are agreeable to this) to reduce the amount of pressure exerted directly on the abdomen (see Chapter 9). Longer term management involves the use of a pelvic floor re-training programme as for any other form of stress incontinence. Sexual contact is in fact an extremely good opportunity for a woman to determine whether or not she is using the correct muscles when exercising her pelvic floor. Assuming both partners are willing to discuss the matter the woman can practise the exercises and can receive feedback from her partner who will need to have his fingers, or his penis, inserted into her vagina and also be aware of the muscles which the woman should not be using, particularly the abdominal muscles. This will not only provide accurate feedback to the woman but may also in the long term increase the sexual pleasure for both parties. Such pleasure may, in itself, serve as an added factor to further motivate the individual to persevere with a programme of pelvic floor exercises.

Regular exercising of the pelvic floor is perhaps the ideal area where health education and health promotion can be applied to the field of continence promotion. It has been recognized that regular exercise in general, and pelvic floor exercises in particular, can prevent the onset of stress incontinence. As a result of this it would be wise to include the concept of pelvic floor training in all health education programmes, particularly those related to women's health but not ignoring the need for men to be included in the target group.

REFERENCES AND FURTHER READING

Bates, C., Bradley, W., Glen, E. *et al.* (1975) First Report of the Standardisation of Terminology of Lower Urinary Tract Function. *Scandinavian Journal of Urology and Nephrology* (1977), **11**, 193–6.

Gordon, H. and Logue, M. (1985) Perineal muscle function after childbirth. *The Lancet*, July, **2**(8447), 123–5.

Jonasson, A., Larsson, B. and Pschera, H. (1989) Testing and Training of the pelvic floor muscles after childbirth. *Acta. Obstet. Gynecol. Scand.*, **68**, 301–304.

Laycock, J. (1987) Graded exercises for the pelvic floor muscles in the treatment of urinary incontinence. *Physiotherapy*, **73**, 371–3.

Norton, C. (1986) *Nursing for Continence*, Beaconsfield Press, Beaconsfield.

Peattie, A. and Plevnik, S. (1988) Cones versus physiotherapy as conservative management of genuine stress incontinence. *Proceedings International Continence Society*, **7**(3).

Plevnik, S. (1985) New method for testing and strengthening of pelvic floor muscles. *Proceedings International Continence Society* (London), 267–8.

Sleep, J. and Grant, A. (1987) Pelvic floor exercises in post-natal care. *Midwifery*, **3**, 158–64.

Thomas, T., Plymat, K., Blannin, J. and Meade, T. (1980) Prevalence of urinary incontinence. *British Medical Journal*, **281**, 1243–5.

6

Dribbling and difficulty in voiding

Dribbling and difficulty in voiding are problems which may be associated with two main underlying conditions which generally require different forms of management. The first and most common of these is some form of obstruction to the flow of urine from the bladder and the second is atonic bladder, or an inability of the detrusor muscle to contract.

OUTFLOW OBSTRUCTION

There are two common reasons for outflow obstruction firstly obstruction resulting from some pathology of the urethra and secondly that arising from benign or malignant prostatic hypertrophy.

Urethral obstruction

Strictures Urethral strictures may be congenital in nature, although this is comparatively rare: they are more commonly associated with scar tissue formation following inflammation or direct trauma (Blandy, 1989). As previously mentioned, inflammation can result from infection or chemical urethritis. Both of these can damage the urethral mucosa resulting in scarring and consequent risk of stricture formation. Direct trauma to the urethra is less common and is only likely to occur if there has been a previous history of catheterization which has led to trauma on insertion or removal of the catheter or the formation of necrotic areas within the urethra resulting from traction or too large a catheter. The other causes of urethral trauma are either direct external force, or insertion of foreign bodies into the urethra, both of which can result in quite severe damage and may in themselves require emergency surgical intervention.

Carcinoma of the urethra   Although this is comparatively rare it should be borne in mind as a possible cause of outflow obstruction.

The problems which a patient will complain of if suffering from a urethral stricture will be very similar to those experienced by a man with prostatic enlargement which are described below.

Prostatic enlargement

Anatomy and physiology   The prostate gland lies just below the bladder neck and above the external sphincter. It surrounds the urethra at this point (the prostatic urethra) and consists of a coiled collection of tubes supported by connective tissue divided into three lobes, one posterior to the urethra and two

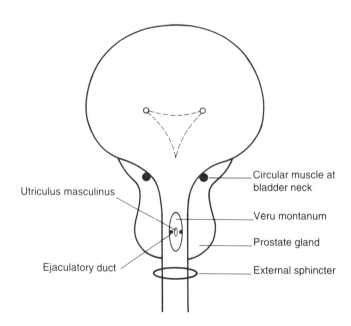

Figure 6.1   Relationship of the prostate gland to the veru montanum.

situated anteriorly and laterally to the urethra. Running through the prostate are the ejaculatory ducts which empty into the urethra at the veru montanum (Figure 6.1).

The function of the prostate is to secrete a comparatively thin milky fluid which is emitted at ejaculation. This fluid contributes approximately 30% of the total ejaculate and has an alkaline pH. This is important if sperm motility is to be maximized since vaginal secretions are normally acidic (pH 3–3.5) and sperm are at their most motile in an environment where the pH is approximately 6–6.5 (Tortora and Anagnostakos, 1990).

Cancer of the prostate   Malignant prostatic enlargement is responsible for 15–20% of cancers in adult males. The most common site for the tumour is the posterior lobe of the prostate and the growth of the tumour is related to the production of androgens, predominantly testosterone, which are produced by the Leydig cells of the testes. Diagnosis is by trans-rectal palpation of the gland which can be felt as a hard nodule, blood serum levels of acid phosphatase, which is raised in cancer of the prostate, and biopsy. It is not uncommon to find that patients who have cancer of the prostate also have a degree of benign hypertrophy as well although there is no evidence to suggest that benign hypertrophy predisposes to malignancy (Watson and Royle, 1992).

Benign prostatic hypertrophy   It has been suggested that all men over the age of 40 will have some degree of prostatic enlargement due to benign hypertrophy but that only 10% of these will experience any degree of obstruction (Blandy, 1989). This, however, is still a significant proportion of the male population and it would appear that benign enlargement is a normal part of the ageing process since no other factors seem to be involved.

URINARY PROBLEMS ASSOCIATED WITH PROSTATIC ENLARGEMENT

Regardless of the cause of the enlargement the problems which a patient experiences as a result of an enlarged prostate are by and large the same and it is these which will usually prompt the man to seek help.

Acute retention of urine

This is perhaps the most dramatic problem which will be encountered in prostatic enlargement since it occurs suddenly and is responsible for producing quite severe discomfort and pain. Although it is usually one of the later problems which a patient with an enlarged prostate is likely to experience it can occur without any prior noticeable or reported urinary problems. The problem is frequently precipitated by over distension of the bladder which often results from the man drinking a few pints of beer and then being unable to find a place to void. When he subsequently attempts to void he finds that he is unable to do so. The outcome of this is that he presents himself at an accident and emergency department usually in severe pain and possibly with some dribbling leakage of urine. The only solution to this is catheterization in order to drain the bladder.

Generally speaking most nurses seem to be in agreement that drainage of the bladder under these circumstances should be performed gradually to avoid the risk of too rapid a release of pressure on the abdominal organs and blood vessels which, in extreme circumstances, may carry a risk of inducing low resistance shock. Once the bladder has been drained the catheter can remain *in situ* for 24–48 hours (Blandy, 1989) and then be removed. The patient is then instructed to attempt to void on an hourly basis initially to ensure that he is capable of doing so. In the majority of cases this period of rest for the bladder will be sufficient to allow a normal pattern of micturition to be re-established and the individual can then be monitored by his GP until he is admitted for surgery. Following an episode of acute retention it is advisable for the man to avoid bouts of excessive fluid intake, and also to continue to void frequently (a two hourly basis is probably adequate) in order to reduce the risk of a further episode of bladder over distension.

A more common presentation of prostatic enlargement is a gradually increasing number of problems associated with voiding. These are described in the following paragraphs.

Hesitancy

As a result of the obstruction and the fact that the detrusor muscle will have to work harder to expel the urine past it the man may complain of great difficulty in starting to void. In some individuals this may be coupled with difficulty in maintaining a steady stream of urine while voiding due to intermittent contraction of the detrusor.

Poor stream

As well as experiencing a 'stop-start' flow of urine the actual force of the urinary stream will be reduced and it is not uncommon for men with prostatic enlargement to urinate on their shoes or down the outside of their trousers as a result of this.

Frequency, urgency and nocturia

These problems are the consequence of incomplete bladder emptying which effectively reduces the functional capacity of the bladder. This also leads to an increased risk of urinary tract infection since the pool of residual urine provides an ideal medium for bacterial growth.

Terminal or post-micturition dribble

The majority of men experience some very slight degree of wetness on their underwear following micturition. This is due to a small amount of urine being held in the urethra as a result of capillary forces. When the meatus comes into contact with clothing the capillary force exerted by this exceeds that in the urethra and the urine is 'sucked' out and absorbed into the cloth. In terminal dribbling the situation is slightly different in that the man feels that he has finished voiding completely, but in fact has not. This leads to a further few millilitres of urine being voided a short time after the main void. Often this is sufficient to cause wetness of the trousers as well as the underwear and can be a source of acute embarrassment to the individual.

This may also occur in some people who do not have a problem with obstruction and is caused by a pooling of urine in

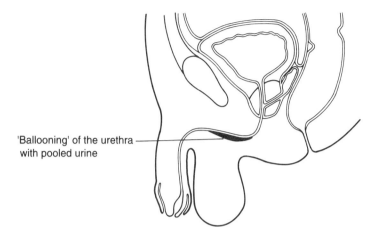

'Ballooning' of the urethra
with pooled urine

Figure 6.2   Enlargement of the urethra allowing pooling of urine.

a slightly enlarged section of the urethra (Figure 6.2). In both
cases the problem can usually be solved by instructing the man
to 'milk' the urethra. This is done by placing two or three
fingers on the perineum behind the scrotum and exerting slight
pressure accompanied by a gentle forward movement. This
forces the urine towards the meatus and the remaining urine
can then be expelled by milking and shaking of the penis.

Many men will suffer the problems associated with prostatic
hypertrophy for several years without seeking help for their
condition. Part of the reason for this is that the problems which
they experience may be very insidious in nature and increase
over this period of time and they become accustomed to living
with them and adapt their lifestyles accordingly. The other
main reason being that there may be a high degree of embarrassment associated with the problem, not least because they
consider that any treatment for it may threaten their ability to
have an erection and to father children thus detracting from
what they perceive to be their 'manhood'. Apart from the
obvious problem which this can create for the nurse in building
up a relationship with the patient, it may also lead to certain
physiological problems for the man.

These problems stem from the fact that if the man has a
chronically distended bladder, as a result of high volumes of

residual urine, the pressure within the bladder is always above normal. This chronic pressure increase, coupled with the fact that there will have been intermittently high pressures as a direct result of the obstruction leading to hypertrophy of the detrusor, can lead to an ultimate weakening of the bladder wall and the formation of bladder diverticula. These further weaken the detrusor muscle causing reduced efficiency of contraction. They are also an ideal site for stone formation and a focus for infection. Further to this the pressure may be sufficiently high to cause reflux of urine into the ureters and ultimately the renal pelvis, which not only increases the risk of upper urinary tract infection, but may also cause hydroureter and hydronephrosis both of which are likely to be irreversible. There may also be a significant effect on the sensory impulses from the bladder. When the bladder is continually distended there is an increased level of sensory output from the trigone. If the individual is unable, or unwilling, to respond to this and fails to empty his bladder the sensory impulses decrease over a period of time and the ability to recognize a full bladder is lost as is the ability to initiate detrusor contraction. This leads to a state of chronic retention of urine accompanied by a dribbling overflow incontinence and the person can be considered to have an atonic bladder. Because this has occurred over a long period of time and the sensory nerves have effectively become desensitized the condition is usually painless, as opposed to acute retention where the sensory tracts remain intact and the individual experiences acute pain.

PHYSIOLOGY OF ATONIC BLADDER

The primary physiological factor leading to atonic bladder is concerned with the sensory nerve pathways leading from the trigone to the spinal cord. If there is a disturbance or disruption to these pathways the person will have reduced or absent sensation of bladder filling. Since stimulation of the motor nerves which cause detrusor contraction and opening of the sphincter is dependent on receiving this sensory impulse their function is also impaired. The consequence of this is that little or no bladder contraction takes place and the sphincter remains closed. Under these circumstances the bladder continues to fill with urine which is contained until the pressure within the bladder exceeds that exerted by the closed sphincter at which point urine begins to leak from the urethra, normally as a fairly constant dribble which may be increased by a rise in intra-abdominal pressure.

Disruption to the sensory pathways may be caused by various factors. As mentioned above, chronic obstruction can lead to a desensitization of the nerve pathways, but this can occur even in the absence of obstruction if an individual constantly ignores the urge to void. In reality this has the same effect as chronic obstruction in that the individual becomes used to having an over distended bladder and only responds to the urge to void when the bladder volume is in excess of normal. Ultimately the sensation of bladder fullness may be lost completely and the person becomes unable to empty their bladder at all. Damage to the sensory nerves as a result of diabetic neuropathy or other degenerative nervous system diseases, low spinal cord lesions at the S2–S4 level and the general deterioration of nervous system and muscle function associated with the ageing process can also lead to the development of atonic or, if the bladder function is not lost entirely, hypotonic bladder (Winder, 1992).

Nursing interventions for outflow obstruction and atonic bladder

In general terms regardless of the cause the aim of care is to prevent or reduce the urinary problems which the person is experiencing even if this is a comparatively short term measure while they are awaiting surgery for an enlarged prostate or urethral stricture.

INTERMITTENT SELF-CATHETERIZATION

Intermittent self-catheterization (ISC) appears to be growing in popularity as a means of managing atonic bladder and as a short term alternative to the use of indwelling catheters for the management of outflow obstruction. As long as the patient has a degree of manual dexterity and is willing to persevere with this technique it is possible to reach a stage where he or she no longer suffers from any episodes of wetness at all. The aim of ISC is to prevent the accumulation of sufficiently large volumes of urine in the bladder to cause overflow incontinence. This not only prevents wetness but also reduces the risk of severe urinary tract infection since the volumes of residual urine which provide an ideal medium for bacterial growth are reduced and the bladder is emptied completely. Despite the fact that ISC is an invasive procedure there is considerably less risk of introducing infection to the urinary tract than is encountered when using indwelling catheters although a number of patients do suffer from an asymptomatic chronic bacteriuria when using this technique and if this becomes problematic then alternative management strategies will have to be considered (Norton, 1986). The other element which may cause some concern regarding ISC is the risk of urethral trauma resulting from repeated catheter insertion. Two factors need to be borne in mind with regard to this. Firstly there is a reduced risk of trauma resulting from traction on the catheter since it is re-moved after each bladder emptying and secondly the catheter is normally being inserted by the individuals themselves and if they are experiencing pain on insertion they are more likely to stop and proceed more gently thus reducing the risk of trauma still further. This may not always be the case when a catheter is being inserted by a nurse or doctor. The use of self-lubricating catheters may also help to ensure that there is an even dis-tribution of lubricant throughout the length of the urethra and hence reduce the risk of trauma at a high level.

Selection of suitable patients for ISC

In purely physiological terms any patient who has overflow incontinence resulting from outflow obstruction, or who suffers from recurrent urinary tract infections as a result of high residual urine volumes, may be a suitable candidate for ISC as long as he or she does not have a completely impassable obstruction in the urethra or some other urethral pathology which could be further aggravated by the frequent passage of a catheter. In real terms however acquiring the skill of ISC requires a high level of motivation on the part of the patient and in most cases a degree of manual dexterity. It is these two factors which may determine whether or not an individual is successful in managing his or her incontinence by this method. Manual dexterity and suppleness may be of particular importance in women who wish to use ISC due to the increased difficulty which they may have in locating the urethral orifice despite the various aids which are available to help overcome this problem. In some cases, if both parties fully understand the implications of the technique and are agreeable, it is possible for the patient's carer to perform the technique although there may be a slightly increased risk of urinary tract infection under these circumstances. This technique is also suitable for children to use, and patient teaching should include them as well as any parent or guardian who may be involved in their care.

Choice of catheter for ISC

Various catheters are available for ISC ranging from single use disposable catheters to rigid catheters which are suitable for sterilization and may last several years. Generally speaking the smallest diameter catheter possible should be used in order to minimize the degree of urethral trauma suffered by the patient. Unlike indwelling catheters the disposable ISC catheters are normally made of PVC. They are also available in different lengths for males and females to allow for the longer urethra in the male. If a chair-bound female is using ISC they may need to use a male length catheter in order to allow for drainage over the edge of the chair. The female catheters are usually more rigid than the male catheters in order to facilitate easier insertion whilst the male catheters must still retain a degree of flexibility to allow their passage along the 'S' shape of the urethra (Figure 6.3). If a woman is having difficulty in locating the urethral orifice special catheters are available which incorporate a mirror on the shaft of the catheter or, alternatively, a catheter guide can be used which helps to locate the catheter in the correct position (Norton, 1993).

Except in hospital, where the risk of cross infection is high, the PVC catheters can be used for up to one week and then replaced and the rigid re-usable catheters used indefinitely and sterilized between use.

The process of ISC

As with all patients suffering from incontinence the first stage of any intervention is to determine when the incontinent episodes occur. In the case of overflow incontinence this in-

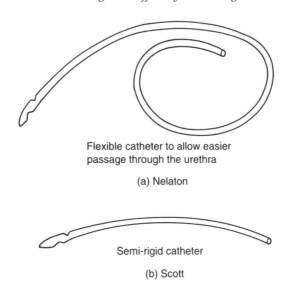

Flexible catheter to allow easier
passage through the urethra

(a) Nelaton

Semi-rigid catheter

(b) Scott

Figure 6.3 Nelaton (male length) and Scott (female length) catheters for intermittent catheterization.

volves establishing a 'leaking' pattern rather than a voiding pattern. That is to say that the time interval between having a completely empty bladder (following drainage via a catheter) and the first signs of dribbling must be determined. This is to ensure that ISC takes place before leakage occurs and is not performed unnecessarily in the interim period. This time will of course vary, depending on fluid intake, but with experience individuals can usually adapt to this and self-catheterize more or less frequently according to circumstances.

When teaching a patient how to self-catheterize, one of the most important aspects to emphasize from the start is that of hygiene. Unlike catheterization in a hospital setting the procedure is considered to be clean as opposed to aseptic but, despite this, attention to hygiene is still of the utmost importance since good hygiene will reduce the risk of urinary tract infection. Hand washing and cleaning and storage of the catheter are probably the two most significant aspects relating to hygiene. It must be stressed to patients that they should wash their hands with soap and water prior to and after each catheterization, and at least rinse the catheter through with running water after use, and preferably wash it with soap followed by a thorough rinse to prevent irritation from residual traces of soap. In some circumstances, such as when using public lavatories, facilities may be lacking and this may not be possible. Because of this it is advisable for anyone who is using ISC to carry disposable wipes for hand cleansing and, whenever possible, to try not to re-use the catheter until they have had the opportunity to wash it.

Storage of the catheter between use is also important and one of the most suitable containers is a self-sealing polythene bag which not only protects the catheter from contamination but is also unobtrusive and easy to carry around in a pocket or handbag. Generally speaking the sequence for performing ISC is as follows:

1. Wash hands.
2. Adopt the position which has been found to be most suitable for the procedure.
3. Insert the catheter until urine begins to flow.
4. When the flow of urine ceases slowly withdraw the catheter.
5. If more urine begins to flow leave the catheter in place until it stops.
6. Withdraw completely.
7. Wash and rinse catheter under running water and replace in storage bag.
8. Wash hands.

This procedure varies somewhat between men and women and the following points need to be included dependent on the sex of the individual.

Men   It is considerably easier for the majority of men to find the urethral meatus than it is for the majority of women. The only exception to this is if a man has a very retracted penis. The most important point for men to remember is that ISC is made easier if the penis is held upright at an angle of approximately 60 degrees to the body. This helps to straighten out the urethral curve and so aid insertion of the catheter. The other important point, particularly if ISC is being carried out in the presence of some form of urethral obstruction, is that the individual should never try to force the catheter if he meets with an unusual level of resistance.

Women   Some women can locate the urethral orifice by touch but most have a degree of difficulty initially. One of the easiest positions for a woman to adopt whilst practising ISC is lying down with her knees bent and her legs apart. This enables her to spread her labia more easily and, if using a mirror to locate the meatus, to see exactly where the catheter is going. Once this has been mastered many women can perform the procedure sitting on the lavatory or standing up with one leg raised resting on the toilet bowl. This, of course, is dependent on their degree of physical ability. One other consideration is that some women find it difficult to perform ISC if they have a tampon *in situ* since this may cause some pressure on the urethra, and they may need to remove it prior to the procedure.

If toilet facilities are unavailable or unsuitable the urine should be drained into some other receptacle and disposed of appropriately. Care should be taken to avoid the catheter coming into contact with the lavatory pan or other receptacle in order to prevent potential contamination from these sources.

Catheter disposal

In a hospital setting catheters should be used once only and then disposed of in the normal manner for potentially contaminated materials which are sent for incineration. In the community catheters should be thoroughly washed in soap and water then sealed in a polythene bag and placed in the dustbin. Although there is minimal risk of infection to others from the catheter, the nurse should check with local infection control officers whether or not there are any special requirements for disposal of catheters used by individuals with infectious diseases.

Anaesthetic and lubricant gels

Initially the use of anaesthetic gel will be helpful for the patient since it will reduce any discomfort which may be experienced. This is true for both sexes although many nurses are under the impression that because of the short length of the female urethra no local anaesthetic is required. This is certainly not universally true and some women can experience severe discomfort when being catheterized or performing ISC (Fowler and Absalom, 1992). If gel is being used it is preferable to have single-use sachets or tubes since once opened the gel is no longer sterile and becomes a potential source of infection. Use of excessive amounts of gel should be discouraged since this leaves a residue in the urethra which again may harbour infection and is pushed up into the bladder at the next catheterization. Once individuals have perfected their technique they may choose to use a water based lubricating gel rather than an anaesthetic gel, or to dispense with gel completely, although the risk of trauma to the urethra should not be forgotten.

Patients should also be advised of certain general considerations which they should take into account when using ISC. These are as follows:

- Fluid intake should be maintained at 1.5–2 litres daily.
- If there are any signs of infection (cloudy smelly urine, a burning sensation in the urethra, pyrexia, etc.) they should increase their fluid intake, take a specimen of urine and attend their GP or clinic.
- Small amounts of blood in the urine or on the catheter may be apparent on occasion, due to minor trauma, but any heavy or persistent bleeding should be reported to their GP as a matter of urgency.

It should also be stressed that catheters should never be cut, and that male patients should not try to use a female length catheter. The danger with this is that if the funnel end has been cut from the catheter it can be inserted too far into the urethra, enter the bladder and then only be removable by cystoscopy, or at worst, open surgery.

ISC is used by some people as the only means of effectively managing their incontinence. Alternatively it can be used as an adjunct to non-invasive voiding techniques if they alone are not sufficient to remove all the residual urine. When used in this way individuals may only need to self-catheterize once or twice a day or less frequently for some people. Indications for this would be recurrent urinary tract infection resulting from residual urine or an abnormally short time interval before leakage occurs when using other techniques.

NON-INVASIVE VOIDING TECHNIQUES

There are two common techniques which can be used to expel urine from an atonic bladder: manual expression or the Crede manoeuvre, and the Valsalva manoeuvre. Both of these rely on an increase in intra-abdominal pressure to force the urine through the sphincter. Neither is likely to be successful if the sphincter is in total spasm, since the pressure which they exert on the bladder, via the abdominal cavity, may be insufficient to overcome the closing pressure of the sphincter.

The Crede manoeuvre

This is achieved by exerting pressure with the ball of the hand above the symphysis pubis. The pressure may be sufficient to produce a bladder spasm, in which case the bladder will empty more or less spontaneously or, if this does not occur, the applied pressure itself can cause voiding to take place. In the latter case the pressure required may be quite considerable, which not only causes discomfort for the person but, in long term use, can also cause damage to the sphincter, leading to stress incontinence and thus complicating the problem. Ureteric reflux will also occur if the pressure within the bladder is raised, and any patients with a history of this, or who complain of loin pain, should be investigated appropriately. It may be necessary for them to use ISC instead.

Valsalva manoeuvre

This is a technique which most people have used at some stage in their lives when trying to pass urine quickly, or if slightly constipated. At its simplest it can be considered as straining. The patient should inhale and then try to exhale whilst blocking the flow of air with the tongue and tensing the abdominal muscles. This produces a rise in intra-abdominal pressure and again, if the sphincter is not in complete spasm, will result in the passage of urine. This procedure is not recommended for any patient who has cardiac problems since, as with any form of straining, it produces stress on the heart, raises the blood pressure and can, in extreme cases, lead to intra-cerebral bleeding or rupture of other blood vessels if there is any underlying weakness. Continual straining of this nature can also lead to weakness of the pelvic floor and the associated problems of stress incontinence and the possibility of faecal incontinence and haemorrhoids.

Techniques for inducing bladder spasm

Some people find that they can induce a bladder spasm without a significant rise in intra-abdominal pressure. Techniques for achieving this are varied and include:

- tapping the abdomen above the symphysis pubis
- pouring cold, or warm, water over the lower abdomen and genitalia
- gentle pulling of the pubic hair
- stroking the cleft between the top of the buttocks
- anal stimulation either by stroking or dilatation.

This is unlikely to be a comprehensive list and individuals may use combinations of the above or have their own technique which they have found to be suitable. Experimentation should be encouraged and any 'new' techniques noted for future reference.

SURGICAL INTERVENTIONS FOR OUTFLOW OBSTRUCTION

Prostatectomy

Since prostatic enlargement is the most common cause of outflow obstruction it follows that this procedure is also the most commonly performed to relieve it.

Trans-urethral resection of the prostate (TURP) The least traumatic approach for prostatectomy is trans-urethrally which does not involve any abdominal incision and is generally followed by a rapid recovery and few urinary problems, as long as the integrity of the external sphincter is maintained. Under normal circumstances potency is maintained.

Retro-pubic prostatectomy This approach is used when the prostate is considered to be too large to remove adequately via the trans-urethral route. It involves an abdominal incision above the symphysis pubis followed by dissection down between the bone and the bladder to reach the prostatic capsule which is opened and the prostatic tissue removed. Again this approach produces a low incidence of post-operative urinary problems and maintains potency. The major disadvantage of this type of surgery is that the recovery time is usually longer than that following trans-urethral prostatectomy due to the presence of an abdominal incision, with the added complication of an incision into the bladder itself.

Trans-vesicle or supra-pubic prostatectomy   This is generally performed only if bladder surgery is indicated as well as prostatic removal, since the approach involves an incision into the bladder through which the prostate is reached. Although urinary results are good and potency is maintained it carries the same problem of an abdominal incision as retro-pubic prostatectomy, with the added complication of an incision in the bladder itself.

Perineal prostatectomy   This is probably the least satisfactory operation since following it the patient may become impotent and have difficulties regaining control of continence.

In general terms, other than in the case of perineal prostatectomy, a patient should have few continence problems following prostatectomy (if the external sphincter remains intact), other than a slight dribbling post-micturition resulting from trauma to the sphincter caused by the catheter. This should resolve quite rapidly and may be improved if the patient performs pelvic floor exercises (and reassurance to this effect should be given). Patients may however experience retrograde ejaculation into the bladder as a result of disruption to the internal sphincter. This needs to be discussed with any patients who are contemplating having children.

Cryosurgery

This is usually performed under local anaesthesia with some degree of sedation. The prostatic tissue is destroyed by using a freezing agent such as liquid nitrogen delivered trans-urethrally via a probe. Post-operatively the patient will require a catheter and care similar to any other post-prostatectomy patient, except there is a lower incidence of haemorrhage when this method is used since the low temperatures involved provide a degree of haemostasis. There are, however, other complications associated with this procedure, including formation of fistulae into the rectum as a result of extensive tissue damage.

Hyperthermia

This is the opposite to the cryosurgery approach in that the prostate is heated by microwaves using either a trans-rectal or trans-urethral approach. It is thought that the action of the heat may be to change the consistency of the glandular tissue as opposed to causing actual shrinkage. Since this is a comparatively new treatment, results to date are inconclusive as to its effectiveness.

Laser treatment

This is carried out under general anaesthetic and the laser beam is directed at the prostatic tissue via a flexible fibre inserted through a cystoscope. The energy produced by the laser serves not only to destroy the prostatic tissue but also to cause coagulation and haemostasis so there is comparatively little blood loss during or following surgery and the need for continuous bladder irrigation is eliminated.

Dilatation of the prostate

This is achieved by the insertion of a catheter with a large inflatable balloon at the tip. Once in position this is inflated so as to stretch the prostate to the point where it splits, thus increasing the lumen of the urethra at this point.

Urethral stents

These consist of a network of plastic or metal strands woven to form a compressed cylinder which, when inserted into the prostatic urethra via a cystoscope, is released and expands thus widening the lumen. Reported success rates for urethral stents are variable: some problems may arise if the stent proves to be ineffective and the patient needs a prostatectomy or replacement stent, since they become integrated with the urethral tissue and may be very difficult to remove.

Urethral stricture

Once diagnosed by cystoscopy this is can be treated surgically by incision of the stricture using a urethrotome and subsequent short term catheterization. Generally this is a successful form of therapy although the risk always remains that new strictures will form as a result of the scar tissue produced. This risk can be significantly reduced by weekly intermittent self-catheterization which keeps the urethra patent.

MANAGEMENT OF OUTFLOW OBSTRUCTION BY LONG TERM INDWELLING CATHETER

In practice any form of urinary incontinence can be managed by the use of long term catheterization, although this should not be considered as first line management due to the problems which are associated with it. The option of this form of management should be discussed fully with patients and their carers.

Problems of long term catheterization

Infection Regardless of the standard of hygiene infection is always a risk if there is a catheter *in situ* since it provides an unobstructed passage directly into the bladder through which pathogens can enter. The first point of infection is during the catheterization procedure itself and this should always be performed using aseptic technique. Following this infection risk can be minimized by using a closed drainage system which prevents ascending infection in the drainage tubes. This is best achieved by reducing the number of times that the catheter itself is disconnected from the drainage bag since all drainage bags should have an integral flutter valve which prevents reflux of urine and bacteria. Because of this, emptying the drainage bag does not in itself constitute a break in the system. There is little need therefore for any special precautions when this is being carried out. Sensible measures however should be taken to avoid gross contamination of the drainage tap such as ensuring that individual catheters are emptied into a sterile or clean jug reserved for that patient and that the end of the tap is not immersed in the urine which has been drained and does not touch the floor. Because of the design of the majority of drainage taps swabbing with alcohol to clean them is a comparatively fruitless activity since it is impossible to ensure contact with all the parts of the tap which have come in contact with the urine. All that is required is that the end of the tap is shaken gently and dried with a tissue to prevent urine spillage on clothing, sheets or the floor. Needless to say hands should be washed before and after emptying each bag and disposable non-sterile gloves should be worn when carrying out the procedure in order to reduce still further the risk of cross infection from nurse to patient and patient to nurse. A further practice which should be adopted is that of changing the drainage bag every 5–7 days as opposed to daily. If the patient has a leg bag a night drainage system should be used where a large volume bag is attached to the tap of the leg bag (still ensuring that there is a non-return valve between the contents of both bags and the bladder).

Risk of discomfort and trauma

As in the case of infection the first stage where discomfort and trauma can occur is during the catheterization process. Insertion of a catheter is a highly skilled procedure and it should only be undertaken by people who have a full knowledge of the anatomy of the urinary tract and have been appropriately trained. If anyone experiences difficulty with catheter insertion, it is preferable to seek advice before continuing rather than exerting force to push the catheter through the urethra. This is most likely to occur in a man with an enlarged prostate, although any form of stricture can cause sufficient resistance to make catheter insertion difficult. As previously mentioned in relation to ISC, the use of anaesthetic gel will greatly reduce the discomfort for the patient and provide lubrication.

The major source of trauma once the catheter is inserted is due to traction on the catheter itself. This can lead to pressure necrosis and ulceration at the bladder neck where the balloon rests and at other points throughout the urethra. In men it is particularly noticeable at the meatus where continued pressure can lead to significant necrosis and splitting of the dorsal surface of the urethra and penis with the consequence that the urethra is laid open. In severe cases this split can extend to the base of the penis causing not only physical but also psychological damage to the patient.

In the majority of patients this sort of trauma can be avoided by paying special attention to securing the catheter to the thigh or clothing with a strip of tape, and ensuring that any drainage bag is adequately supported. Some patients will resist all efforts to achieve this, however, and sit and tug on their catheter to the point where they may pull it out with the balloon still inflated. This can cause gross trauma to the urethra and if attempts to educate the patient with regard to this fail, then it may be necessary to consider an alternative form of management.

Catheter hygiene

Scrupulous hygiene is required when a person has a catheter *in situ* not only to reduce the infection risk but also to prevent discomfort and odour. Even in the absence of infection the majority of patients will experience some discharge around the catheter at the meatus. This is due to increased mucous secretion resulting from irritation of the urethral mucosa by the catheter. The presence of this mucous provides a focus for bacterial growth and, when it hardens, it also has an abrasive action on the urethral membrane causing soreness and ulceration. It is therefore important to clean the catheter at this point at least twice daily, or more frequently if there is excessive secretion. Cleansing should be carried out using disposable gloves and wipes, and soap and water. The catheter should be gently cleaned away from the meatus to avoid forcing soapy water and bacteria up the urethra. Care should be taken not to apply traction to the catheter during this procedure for the reasons described above. In women particularly it may be necessary to perform perineal washing and catheter cleansing after they have had their bowels open due to the proximity of the meatus to the anus. In both sexes, the use of talcum powder or creams around the meatal area should be discouraged, since they can combine with the secretions to form a larger mass, and hence further discomfort for the patient.

Overall the interventions required to promote continence in a person with difficulty in voiding or dribbling incontinence call for a complete review of his or her 'normal' elimination routines. Because of this a high level of patient support is needed to encourage them to persevere with whatever form of management has been decided upon. Despite this the inter-ventions can be almost 100% effective in maintaining con-tinence whether they are used as long term management or in the short term while the patient is awaiting surgery.

REFERENCES AND FURTHER READING

Blandy, J. (1989) *Lecture Notes on Urology*, 4th edn, Blackwell Scientific Publications, Oxford.

Fowler, C. and Absalom, M. (1992) Catheterisation, in *Endoscopic Urology for Nurses* (eds M. Absalom and D. Betts), Academic Unit of Urology (Royal London Hospital), London.

Norton, C. (1986) *Nursing for Continence*, Beaconsfield Press, Bea-consfield.

Norton, C. (1993) A helping handle. *Nursing Times*, **89**(16), 76–8.

Tortora, G. and Anagnostakos, N. (1990) *Principles of Anatomy and Physiology*, 6th edn, Harper and Row, London. Chapter 26.

Watson, J. and Royle, J. (1992) *Medical-Surgical Nursing and Related Physiology*, 4th edn, Baillière Tindall, London. Chapter 23.

Winder, A. (1992) Intermittent Self Catheterisation, in *Clinical Nursing Practice* (ed B. Roe), Prentice Hall, London.

7

Lack of awareness of the need to void

Although a person with an atonic bladder may be unaware of the fact that his or her bladder is full, an alternative situation exists whereby an individual has little or no sensation of a full bladder. Unlike the situation with atonic bladder, however, there is no disturbance to the sensory pathways from the bladder; therefore voiding can still take place. This occurs if there is damage to the spinal nerve pathways above the level of S2, dysfunction of the cerebral micturition control centre or if there is a degree of mental impairment which prevents an individual from recognizing the appropriate time or place to void, as occurs in acute and chronic confusional states and in some people with learning difficulties.

REFLEX BLADDER EMPTYING

If there is damage to the nerve pathways between the reflex arc level of the spinal cord (S2–S4) the message that the bladder is filling cannot be transmitted to the brain. The net result of this is that bladder function returns to that which is found in babies in that, when the bladder is full, the sensory impulse from it triggers the reflex arc to initiate the motor signals which cause sphincteric relaxation and detrusor contraction in the absence of any cerebral control or inhibition. A similar pattern occurs if there is damage to, or dysfunction of, the cerebral control centre, as may occur in cerebro-vascular accident and some other brain disorders. In both these cases the individual will experience a full and uncontrollable void with no prior warning that it is about to occur.

Management of reflex bladder emptying

The exact management of reflex emptying is dependent on the cause of the problem. Management techniques will vary in order to cater for individuals who have experienced acute illness or trauma, and can therefore be divided into short and long term phases.

Short term management

This will vary in detail depending on the cause of the problem. If the patient has been spinally injured there is likely to be a period of time during which nervous system function is so severely disrupted that the normal reflex function of the spinal cord is also absent (Watson and Royle, 1992). This may also occur in the case of cerebro-vascular disease and head injury. During this phase the person is likely to suffer retention of urine and it may be desirable to consider indwelling catheterization or possibly intermittent catheterization in order to maintain dryness. Although intermittent catheterization can be considered to be preferable to the use of an indwelling catheter the patient's general condition must be taken into account and consideration given as to the amount of disturbance which ISC may cause to the patient since excessive stimulation may lead to cerebral irritation and aggravate what is already a potentially unstable condition (Jennett and Teasdale, 1981). Other factors may also impinge on this such as the presence of other injuries. If the damage is traumatic, these must be taken into account. What is perhaps most important to remember is that the catheterization should only be planned as a short term measure and that other approaches should be considered as soon as the patient's condition allows. Following this period of nervous system inactivity the reflex function of the spinal cord should normally begin to reappear. This will occur within a few days of the initial trauma, and it is at this point that removal of the catheter must be considered and a longer term management plan drawn up.

Long term management

Once the catheter has been removed the patient needs close observation to ensure that any signs of retention are noted early and acted upon. This may necessitate re-catheterization but again this should only be regarded as a short term solution. All being well, the patient will begin to void spontaneously. Due to the reduced mobility which many of these patients experience it is essential to ensure that they are attended to promptly, and washed and dried in order to reduce the risk of skin excoriation and pressure sore formation. In the case of male patients a urinary sheath may be a useful aid during this period whilst pads will be necessary for females. As with any other form of incontinence it is important to maintain an accurate record of when the patient voids. This is the basis for further management of the problem, since the emptying of a bladder which is functioning on a reflex is dependent upon a certain volume of urine being reached which is sufficient to produce the sensory impulses to trigger the reflex arc at the spinal cord. If frequency/volume records are kept it is likely that not only will the timing of bladder emptying show a distinct pattern but also that the volume of urine voided each time will be approximately the same. This is particularly true if the person's fluid intake is regulated to try to ensure that roughly the same volumes of fluid are consumed at the same times each day.

Once the pattern has been established incontinent episodes can be avoided by toileting the patient at the appropriate time. Alternatively, if individuals are able, they can toilet themselves by whatever means they can manage. Voiding can often be prompted in these circumstances by slight abdominal pressure or tapping as in the case of atonic bladder. If this is done long waits in the toilet can be reduced and a more normal life can be led although individuals may still choose to use pads or a sheath for added security and at night. Over a period of time most people who use this method of management reduce the number of episodes of wetness considerably as a result of becoming familiar with the various factors which affect their rate of urine production. It may help if these are discussed in broad terms with patients at quite an early stage so that they can begin to observe them for themselves. The other point to remember is that although an individual may have no bladder sensation as such, the pressure from the bladder is transferred to other abdominal organs. Many people will be able to detect this and can then use it, in conjunction with an individualized timed toileting programme, to predict when their bladder is nearing the point when it will contract and hence further reduce the risk of incontinent episodes. This technique can also be used for unconscious patients and may in fact carry even less risk of wetness since the fluid intake is normally more controlled. Patients who are unconscious will obviously not be able to toilet themselves and it is up to the nursing staff to ensure that a urinal or bedpan is provided at the appropriate time. Again gentle abdominal pressure or tapping may prompt a void which will reduce the length of time it takes for an individual to be successfully toileted. In some people, the bladder contraction which results from this reflex emptying may not be sufficient to expel all of the urine present, and the amount of residual urine may be comparatively high. If this is suspected, the situation should be investigated by passing a catheter postvoid or by using abdominal ultrasound. The problems which are associated with incomplete bladder emptying are no less significant for this group of people than for those with outflow obstruction and it may be necessary for people with a high residual urine to use intermittent self-catheterization (see Chapter 6) as an adjunct to the timed toileting, albeit less often than if they were completely unable to void. Strictly speaking the use of ISC as a first line management for a reflex bladder is also a possible option and may be preferred by some patients. It must be remembered, however, that there are potential complications associated with ISC and it may not ultimately produce any better results than a toileting programme; thus the complications could outweigh any advantages.

INABILITY TO RECOGNIZE THE APPROPRIATE TIME AND/OR PLACE TO VOID

The appropriateness of places to void may be open to some interpretation since it may vary considerably between cultures and settings. Regardless of this it is usually apparent when an individual is voiding inappropriately within their own cultural setting.

The most common cause of inappropriate voiding within this category is some form of altered mental state. Although this is generally considered to be associated with a form of confusion, be it acute or chronic, it is not unreasonable to extend the concept of altered mental state to drug induced confusion (including that induced by alcohol) and even to the state of sleep and nocturnal enuresis.

Confusional states

These are most commonly associated with the elderly who are suffering from some form of dementia such as Alzheimer's disease or multi-infarct dementia. The common manifestation of this in relation to incontinence is as follows.

Inability to find/remember where the toilet is　Anyone with severe memory problems may experience this problem. They do not appear necessarily to have lost the sensation of the need to void, and will often get up and wander around the house, or ward apparently looking for something. It may even be that by the time they have found the toilet, if they are able to find it, they have forgotten exactly what they wanted to do in the first place. More frequently they are unable to find the toilet and either void in a wholly inappropriate place (such as the middle of the room) or try to find a substitute such as a bucket, chair or any other receptacle which is available. The classic nursing response to this is the use of some form of reality orientation (Duffy, 1990) whereby the individual is reminded of where the toilet is, what it is for and if necessary how it should be used. This approach is accompanied by clearly visible signposts to the toilet often using some form of pictorial representation to further emphasize exactly where the toilet is situated. For some people this will be sufficient stimulus to prevent, or at least significantly reduce, the incidence of incontinence, but for many others its effect remains unnoticeable.

INABILITY TO EXPRESS THE NEED TO VOID

This may be the result of a confusional state or an expressive dysphasia. Regardless of the cause the major nursing problem in this situation is that the individuals are unable to tell their carers what they need and also in many cases unable to co-operate with any regime which is planned. Here again it is of vital importance to establish whether there is a pattern to the incontinence and, if there is, to implement an individualized toileting programme.

It must be emphasized at this point that this does not mean two hourly toileting – a practice which is unfortunately widespread in a number of hospital wards and other care settings, and which is often the only attempt made to control incontinence. Two hourly toileting tends to be based on nursing routines and convenience rather than on patient need. It is also responsible for wasting a lot of nursing time and for a potential increase in the number of incontinent episodes experienced by the patients (Southern and Henderson, 1990). The vast majority of people do not void on a two hourly basis and even if they are taken to the toilet it is unlikely that someone who has reduced awareness and/or nervous system function will be sufficiently competent to void voluntarily. This leads to the situation whereby an individual who has been taken to the toilet, and not used it, can then be left for a further two hours, during which time he or she may well have voided spontaneously. Not only is this a waste of time but it is also inappropriate care based on routine rather than on an individualized plan. Two hourly toileting regimes should only be implemented if this is the pattern which has been identified for a specific individual as a result of assessment and the use of a continence chart. The other factor to remember is that a number of patients, although unable to inform their carers of the need to void and unable to take themselves to the toilet, will be aware themselves of the need to void and exhibit tell tale signs of this ranging from restlessness to outright aggression. A skilled nurse who knows his or her patients will be able to recognize these signs and act on them accordingly. Any information of this nature should also be sought at the assessment stage and documented appropriately in patients' nursing records.

BEHAVIOURAL INCONTINENCE

Exactly what can be classed as behavioural incontinence is open to debate since the term may be used to refer to problems a patient is experiencing as described above, or alternatively may imply some form of intent (be it conscious or unconscious) on the part of the individual concerned, i.e. some form of attention seeking. This may be a dangerous and inappropriate label to apply to a patient, since what is perceived as attention seeking behaviour by the nurse may, in fact, be the result of a genuine inability to control voiding on the part of the patient. It is likely that some patients are labelled as attention seeking and accused of 'doing it on purpose' simply because of a lack of knowledge or thought on the part of the nursing staff in relation to the other potential causes of incontinence. Having said this there is little doubt that certain patients do appear to wet themselves in order to gain attention from their carers, since once wet they can be assured, at some stage, of receiving at least a few minutes of nursing time. Often all that is required in this situation is some form of diversionary therapy which keeps the individual's mind occupied and/or meets the need for social interaction. This may be easier said than done in a ward situation where nursing staff can be fully occupied with attending to the physical needs of their patients. Equally difficult is the community setting where a carer has to go out to work, or leave the person alone for long periods of time.

Such a situation is sometimes identifiable when a person is admitted to hospital with a comparatively short history of incontinence which resolves spontaneously when he or she begins to interact with the ward staff and other patients.

If perceived isolation appears to be the cause of a person's incontinence then it is essential that all avenues are explored, including voluntary and statutory agencies which may be in a position to offer help and support both in a hospital and community setting. It may be desirable to initiate some form of behaviour modification programme whereby the person receives attention and praise for being continent which outweighs the attention received when he or she is incontinent. This is not to say that individuals who fail to become continent, despite extra attention, should be censured for it, rather that incontinent episodes should be attended to with the minimum of fuss and in the quickest time possible while still ensuring that the care which is required is actually given. In this way such patients may come to recognize that continence is preferable to incontinence and that they receive a 'better quality' of attention if they remain dry (Norton, 1986).

DRUG INDUCED INCONTINENCE

Diuretics are not the only drugs which may be associated with causing a person to become incontinent. In reality any drug which alters the mental state of an individual – such as tranquillizers, night sedation and, most commonly, alcohol – can lead a person to become incontinent or at least suffer from some incontinent episodes. One of the first things which should be considered when individuals are incontinent is their drug therapy, particularly if they have no previous history of incontinence prior to commencing the medications. One very common scenario is of the person who is fully continent during the day but is incontinent at night. All too often this is not fully investigated and is managed by the use of penile sheaths, or pads, without any consideration being given as to whether the person is taking night sedation, or has a high alcohol consumption prior to going to bed. Both of these may be significant factors in causing nocturnal incontinence and may also be difficult problems to overcome. In the case of night sedation the need for it should be discussed with the patient and the doctor and an attempt made to reduce its use with the ultimate goal of complete withdrawal. This can create a number of anxieties for the patient since there may not only be a degree of physical dependence on the drug but also a high level of psychological dependence. Both of these must be addressed and appropriate support given if a successful outcome is to be achieved. If the individual is still incontinent at night after sedation has been withdrawn, then alternative causes for the incontinence should be considered.

Not uncommonly the first time a person receives night sedation is on admission to hospital. The reason for this is usually attributed to the difficulties they may have in adapting to a hospital environment and getting to sleep. Although the importance of sleep cannot be minimized this must be balanced with the potential problems of introducing a person to a drug which may lead to dependence and other associated problems. Responsibility for this lies partly with the prescribers and partly with the nursing staff who administer the medication. It would appear that this problem is particularly relevant to the elderly about whom various assumptions are made when they are admitted to hospital. Firstly it is assumed that they will require some form of analgesia, secondly that they will be suffering from constipation and thirdly that they will need night sedation, regardless of whether they have taken it at home. These are duly prescribed in the 'as required' section of the patient's drug chart with the consequence that night sedation in particular may be routinely offered to patients simply because they have been written up for it, with no regard as to whether they actually need it. This may lead to incontinence with an increased risk of falls during the night if a person does wake and attempt to get out of bed, neither of which reflect high standards of care.

Alcohol consumption is perhaps a more difficult problem to tackle since it may only take a comparatively small amount of alcohol to induce a deep sleep in some individuals whereas others may be drinking what could be considered excessive amounts. In the former case, discussion with the patient about whether alcohol may be the cause of the incontinence may be sufficient to lead him or her to reconsider drinking before going to sleep, and the problem can be resolved in this manner. Excessive alcohol consumption on the other hand may be indicative of addiction and an underlying alcohol problem. The management of this requires specialist assessment and intervention and in itself falls outside the remit of continence promotion which can only be realistically attempted after the underlying difficulties have been resolved.

NOCTURNAL ENURESIS

This is a problem primarily associated with children and young adults although it can occur in older people either as a continuation of a lifelong problem for which they have not sought any help, or as a problem which has developed in later life (Brocklehurst, 1984). Regardless of when the problem starts the difficulties which it can cause in terms of extra washing, embarrassment and tension within relationships are immense and it is therefore a significant area where the nurse can be involved.

Physiological basis for nocturnal enuresis

The prime physiological element in relation to nocturnal enuresis is the ability of the brain to subconsciously recognize that the bladder is full and rouse the individual from their sleep in order to go to the toilet. If the sleep is so deep that this stimulus is not recognized or acted upon then the inhibitory effect of the micturition control centre ceases to act and the bladder empties. In some people sleep may be so deep that they still do not wake even when they are wet. In direct contrast to this is the situation whereby an individual is aware of having a full bladder but is dreaming of actually being in the toilet and thus being free to pass urine without any problem. This frequently occurs when individuals are sleeping comparatively lightly and in most cases they wake either just before they are about to void or very rapidly when they have only passed a few millilitres of urine, at which point they are able to control the void until they can reach the toilet. This group of people generally only experience occasional incontinent episodes and have fewer problems with it than those who void a bladderful.

If someone is experiencing nocturnal enuresis, regardless of their age, there are two main approaches that can be adopted. The first, like so many others related to continence promotion, relies on determining whether or not there is a pattern to the person's bed-wetting. If it is established that the person wets the bed at approximately the same time each night, an alarm clock can be set to wake him or her shortly before this would normally occur. This then allows the person to exercise conscious control over bladder emptying until the toilet can be reached. If an individual is not woken by an alarm, or has a hearing impairment, a vibrating pad under the pillow is a suitable alternative to an alarm clock.

If no pattern can be established then the use of an enuresis alarm should be considered (Figure 7.1). The basic principle of these is that when someone wets the bed a low voltage, battery operated, electrical circuit is completed and the alarm sounds and wakes the person. Again, if an individual is hard of hearing, or shares a room with others who would be disturbed by the alarm, a vibrating pad may be used. Once wakened it is possible for patients to again exercise conscious control over their voiding and reduce the amount of urine lost over a period of time with the ultimate goal of wakening before wetting the bed at all or ideally sleeping through the night without needing to void. There is little doubt that this form of conditioning can

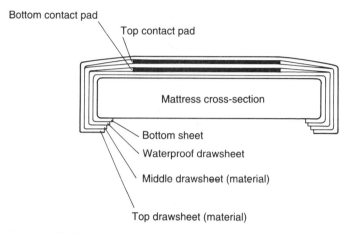

Figure 7.1 Basic enuresis alarm.

be very successful in 'sensitizing' the sleeping brain to the messages which it receives from the bladder and leading the individual either to wake when the bladder is full, or to exercise greater inhibitory control whilst asleep, leading to a less disturbed night.

Psychological factors in nocturnal enuresis

It has been identified that the onset or recurrence of nocturnal enuresis is often associated with some form of stress, which is often unrecognized or unacknowledged (Meadow and Smithells, 1986). This may be within a home setting or it could be due to factors outside the home such as school, exams or work. In extreme cases it may also lead to daytime incontinence.

Under these circumstances the use of an enuresis alarm may prove to be comparatively fruitless since the problem is not primarily physiological and may require in-depth intervention by a psychologist. Psychological elements should always be considered when a person is being assessed and it is important to recognize any cues which may be given by individuals or parents which could give some indication of potential stressors. A high degree of sensitivity is required in order to try to elicit sufficient information to allow meaningful discussion of the problem to take place and to introduce the possibility of referral to a psychologist since this could be perceived as a very threatening step by some individuals.

If it is found that the use of an enuresis alarm, with or without appropriate psychological intervention, is unsuccessful the problem can be managed by the use of penile sheaths, pads or washable undersheets (see Chapter 9), all of which if used sensibly can significantly reduce the impact of nocturnal enuresis, both on the individuals concerned and on their carers.

Although many of the individuals who are incontinent as a result of a lack of awareness may appear to fall into the category of 'intractably' incontinent, the fact is that in the majority of cases the nursing interventions which are required are comparatively straightforward and simple. Perhaps one of the most important aspects to remember in relation to this group is that of pattern identification and individualized toileting which is often the only means of achieving a satisfactory result and keeping the individual dry.

REFERENCES AND FURTHER READING

Brocklehurst, J. (1984) *Ageing, Bladder Function and Incontinence: Urology in the Elderly*, Churchill Livingstone, Edinburgh.

Duffy, E. (1990) Helping caregivers cope: managing urinary incontinence associated with Alzheimer's disease. *Journal of Enterostomal Therapy*, **17**, 87–93.

Jennett, B. and Teasdale, G. (1981) *Management of Head Injuries*, F.A. Davis, Philadelphia.

Meadow, S. and Smithells, R. (1986) *Lecture Notes on Paediatrics*, 5th edn, Blackwell Scientific Publications, Oxford.

Norton, C. (1986) *Nursing for Continence*, Beaconsfield Press, Beaconsfield.

Southern, D. and Henderson, P. (1990) Tackling incontinence. *Nursing Times*, **86**(10), 36–8.

Watson, J. and Royle, J. (1992) *Medical-Surgical Nursing and Related Physiology*, 4th edn, Baillière Tindall, London.

8

Faecal incontinence

Despite the fact that faeces are generally considered to be more offensive in nature than urine, faecal incontinence receives less attention than urinary incontinence in nursing texts. The reasons for this are twofold. Firstly the incidence of reported faecal incontinence is lower than that for urinary incontinence (approximately 1% of the population – Thomas, Egan and Meade, 1985), and secondly, unless a person is suffering from diarrhoea, faeces is usually more easily contained within pads than urine, with the consequence that there is less leakage and hence arguably less of a problem with its management. This of course does not lessen the impact on the individual who is experiencing the problem, or on the carers.

ANATOMY AND PHYSIOLOGY OF THE LOWER GASTROINTESTINAL TRACT

For the purposes of this chapter the most significant section of the gastrointestinal tract is the large intestine, rectum and anus. The large intestine in the adult is approximately 1.5 m long and runs from the ileo-caecal valve at the junction of the terminal ileum to the anus. The diameter of the intestine is variable, but on average it is 6–7 cm. It consists of the ascending, transverse and descending colon which constitute the bulk of the organ with the sigmoid colon and rectum making up the terminal portion of the large intestine (Figure 8.1).

The musculature of the large intestine consists of an inner layer of circular muscle surrounded by a layer of longitudinal muscle, parts of which are organized into three distinct bands known as the *taeniae coli*. These stretch for almost the whole

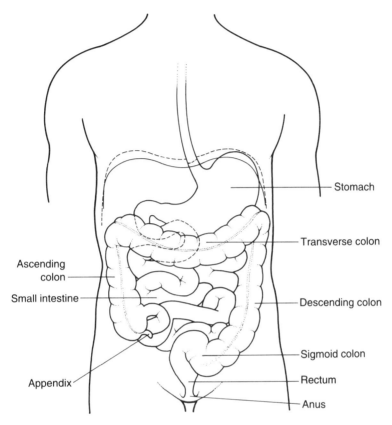

Figure 8.1 Gross anatomy of the large intestine.

length of the large intestine. When they contract the colon is shortened which results in the formation of pouches, or haustra, which give it its characteristic appearance. The musculature allows for peristalsis to take place accompanied by a process known as haustral churning which involves sequential passage of chyme from one haustrum to the next. There is also a process of mass peristalsis which commences at approximately the middle area of the transverse colon and is responsible for providing the impetus to force the contents of the descending colon into the rectum. This form of persistalsis is initiated by the presence of food in the stomach and the duodenum and is the result of the gastrocolic and duodenocolic reflexes which

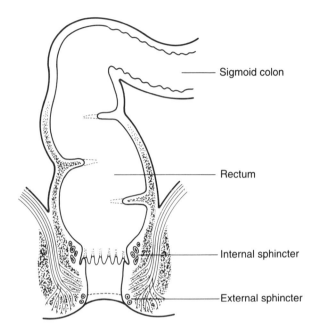

Figure 8.2 Rectum and anal sphincters.

are stimulated when food reaches the stomach and the duodenum. The inner layer of the large intestine consists predominantly of columnar epithelium and goblet cells whose prime functions are absorption of water and secretion of mucous respectively. The sphincter mechanism of the anus consists of an internal sphincter which is under autonomic control and an external sphincter under voluntary control (Figure 8.2).

The formation of faeces and the process of defecation

Despite a high level of water reabsorption taking place in the small intestine the chyme which passes into the colon is comparatively liquid in nature and further reabsorption needs to take place for semi-solid faeces to be formed. This consists of some water, mucous and sloughed epithelial cells from the lining of the gut, salts, bacteria and undigested food. Once the faeces have reached the rectum, pressure receptors in the walls of the rectum initiate the defecation reflex. When distended the receptors send sensory messages to the sacral spinal cord which in turn relays motor impulses to the descending colon, including the rectum itself, and the anus. This then causes a further increase in pressure in the rectum, forcing open the internal sphincter. At this point defecation is controlled by the action of the voluntary external sphincter. If defecation is consciously inhibited the faeces are backed up into the sigmoid colon and the urge to defecate ceases until the next mass peristalsis forces the faeces back into the rectum. If on the other hand the external sphincter is voluntarily relaxed defecation takes place. The processes involved in the voluntary aspects of defecation are similar to those employed in the control of bladder emptying and, as with urinary continence, is a learned response.

Age changes in the large intestine

As with the urinary system there are certain changes which take place in relation to defecation as a part of the normal ageing process. These are primarily related to a loss of muscle tone and strength which may result in a delayed passage of faeces through the colon and a decreased neuronal sensitivity which slows or inhibits the defecation reflex. The final result of these is an increased tendency to constipation, a greater need to strain at stool and the subsequent development of diverticular disease and haemorrhoid formation.

ASSESSMENT IN FAECAL INCONTINENCE

As with urinary incontinence it is vitally important to carry out this stage of the nursing process as comprehensively as possible. Many of the elements which need to be included in this assessment are common with those which should be addressed in an assessment related to urinary incontinence. There are, however, certain additional considerations which should be included. These are as follows.

Normal bowel pattern

It is important to establish the individual's normal defecation pattern and to ascertain the length of time for which the problem has been apparent. This is particularly significant since a change in bowel pattern may be indicative of an underlying neoplasm which must always receive further medical investigation.

Nature of the faeces

Two common causes of faecal incontinence are constipation and diarrhoea. A constipated stool will appear dry and hard and is therefore comparatively easy to recognize. Diarrhoea on the other hand may be the result of a genuinely liquid stool or alternatively the result of impacted faeces and an overflow of liquid stool around the obstruction. It is important to establish whether this is the case since the management of the two conditions differs significantly. Rectal examination at the very least should be performed in order to ascertain whether there are hard faeces in the rectum. Ideally this should be accompanied by radiological investigations since the obstruction is frequently in the colon itself and is only detectable on x-ray.

Any blood or excessive mucous in the faeces should also be investigated by the medical team, since this may be indicative of neoplastic changes.

Faecal odour   Although it is difficult to define exactly what constitutes an offensive smelling stool, it is comparatively easy to recognize a stool which has an odour different to that which could be considered as normal. One factor which must be taken into account when considering the smell of the faeces is the person's diet since this can have a significant effect on the smell. It is important to ask individual patients whether they have noticed any change themselves. Particularly malodourous stools may result from infection or malabsorptive disorders.

Warning of the need to defecate

As with urinary incontinence, the time which different individuals have between recognizing that they have a full rectum and a strong desire to defecate can be very variable. Some people may have lost the sensation completely, either as a result of trauma or degenerative changes in the nervous system, whilst others, particularly if suffering from constipation, may have a permanent feeling that they need to have their bowels open.

Mental awareness

This relates to the ability of the individual to recognize an appropriate time and place to defecate.

In the case of faecal incontinence it is perhaps easier to consider the problems which a patient may be experiencing under the broad headings of 'constipation', 'diarrhoea', 'sphincter weakness' and 'mental state' within which various sub-categories can be identified.

CONSTIPATION

Contrary to popular interpretation, the term constipation does not refer to a complete inability to pass faeces which is more correctly known as obstipation. Constipation merely refers to the passage of hard, dry stools which cause individuals to experience difficulty, often accompanied by pain, when attempting to have their bowels open (Glanze, 1986). Generally the passage of the stools is also considered to be infrequent, but applying this rigidly may lead to some confusion since it is possible for someone who is constipated to be almost constantly passing small quantities of faeces.

Causes of constipation

Broadly constipation can be categorized into two main divisions: rectal constipation or dyschezia where there is a mass of hard faeces collected in the rectum, or colonic constipation where the faecal material is delayed in its passage through the colon and the main collection can be found in the colon itself. In general terms the common causes of constipation are equally applicable to both types, although the interventions required differ.

General causes of constipation Factors such as dietary and fluid intake are perhaps the most significant factors when considering the causes of constipation. A diet which is low in fibre can lead to a low bulk of faeces which is not propelled adequately through the colon leading to an increased transit time (the time which it takes for the gut contents to reach the rectum and be expelled) and a consequent increase in water reabsorption in both the small and large intestine resulting in the production of hard faeces. Equally an inadequate fluid intake may lead to the same result since there is less water to be reabsorbed in the first place. The other general factor which needs to be taken into consideration with regard to transit time is that of the person's mobility. It is likely that a decrease in overall mobility also leads to an increase in transit time (Watson and Royle, 1992).

Drug induced constipation

Perhaps the most common drugs associated with the onset of constipation are the opiate analgesics which can, under certain circumstances, even be used to treat intractable diarrhoea. The action of these, and to a lesser extent of the majority of analgesics, is to reduce gut motility and increase transit time thus increasing water reabsorption and reducing the fluid content of the faeces (Trounce and Gould, 1990). Other drugs which have a similar effect are those which have a direct action on the parasympathetic nervous system, such as anti-cholinergic drugs and several of the antidepressant drugs which have anti-cholinergic side effects.

Excessive laxative use is also frequently implicated as a predisposing factor to the development of constipation in later life. Many people, particularly the elderly, have been brought up to believe that they should have a bowel action at least on a daily basis and, in some cases, an additional 'clear out' at least once a week. In order to achieve this, laxatives have been used, often on a daily basis, with the consequence that the bulk of the faeces in the colon has been reduced. This can have a significant effect on the motility of the gut since peristaltic movement is dependent to a large extent on stimulation of the myenteric reflex. This stimulation only occurs if there is sufficient distension of the bowel by faeces. In the absence of this distension, as occurs if stool softening laxatives are used or if the diet is low in fibre, the reflex is not stimulated and peristaltic action is reduced. In the long term this results in a de-sensitization of the reflex coupled with a decrease in the muscle tone of the gut leading to the development of what is commonly referred to as a 'lazy bowel'.

Neurological causes of constipation

Any neurological condition which affects the sensory and/or motor nerves of the gut can lead to constipation. This includes spinal cord trauma and degenerative neurological conditions such as multiple sclerosis and Parkinson's disease where sufferers have a very high incidence of constipation.

Loss of, or decrease in, the sensitivity of the bowel may also be associated with a chronic tendency to retain faeces and flatus voluntarily. As with other sensory impulses, continued disregard of the 'call to stool' may result in the ultimate loss of sensitivity and consequent problems with constipation. A common reason which is given for ignoring the urge to defecate is the lack of privacy in public lavatories, and in institutional settings, coupled with a fear of embarrassment that someone else will be able to hear and smell what the person is doing. Ano-rectal disorders, such as haemorrhoids, may also lead individuals to reduce the frequency with which they open their bowels in order to avoid any pain which they may experience as a result of the condition.

The other main cause of constipation which should always be considered is the presence of some form of new growth of the bowel. This tends to result in a relatively acute change in a person's bowel habits, often leading to similar feelings of discomfort to those experienced when a person is constipated. These feelings are normally accompanied by constipation, diarrhoea or an alternation between the two. Any changes such as these which are reported by the patient should obviously be investigated fully by the medical team.

FAECAL INCONTINENCE RELATED TO CONSTIPATION

Regardless of the cause of the constipation there are two fundamental reasons why a person may become incontinent if constipated. The first of these is associated with rectal constipation where the impacted faeces are to be found predominantly in the rectum and anal canal. In this case the individual may complain of a constant feeling of having a full rectum and the need 'to go'. Hard impacted faeces will also be palpable on rectal examination. In this situation the patient may be passing small amounts of faeces at frequent intervals, if not all the time. This results from the pressure of the faeces in the rectum forcing faecal matter through the anal sphincter. It is not uncommon for the individual to be unaware of this either as a result of loss of sensitivity, or simply because they have become used to a degree of discomfort, and the actual passage of the faeces does not make a significant difference to this.

Management of this type of incontinence is aimed at preventing the constipation whenever possible. Initially it is essential to clear the faeces which are already present in the bowel. If the stool is hard and impacted it may be necessary to initiate this process by using manual evacuation of the bowel. This should not, however, be undertaken by anyone who is untrained in the technique since it is not only very uncomfortable for the patient but also carries the risk of causing direct trauma to the bowel itself. Softer impacted faeces may be easier for the patient to pass without this procedure being resorted to and usually respond well to the introduction of phosphate enemas. It must be remembered that even if a 'good result' is obtained following the first enema it should not be assumed that all the faeces have been expelled and further enemas may need to be administered on a daily basis, or every two days, until the rectum is fully cleared of the faecal mass. Failure to do this will result in a rapid reoccurrence of the incontinence and the risk that the patient will be labelled as suffering from an intractable condition which can only be managed by the use of occasional enemas and pads, whereas in reality it is the result of inadequate intervention in the first instance. Once the bowel is cleared, the emphasis must be on prevention of constipation. Despite comparatively widespread information on what constitutes a 'healthy diet' in terms of fibre consumption and fluid intake many people, especially the elderly who have been used to eating what they want to for several years, are reluctant to modify their diets to accommodate their changed needs. Here the role of the nurse as a health educator is of paramount importance in stressing the need to adapt a diet which may appear to the individual concerned to be wholly adequate. Personal preferences are not the only obstacles to the success of this type of intervention since a healthy diet may also have some financial implications which the person is unable to meet.

Involvement of the dietitian and, if necessary, the medical social worker may go some way to solving the problem – as may involvement of the family or partner.

With or without a change in dietary habits it may still be necessary for the individual to have some form of laxative medication to promote normal bowel emptying and possibly regular administration of enemas on a weekly or twice weekly basis. When the initial faecal mass has been cleared using phosphate enemas it may be possible to use suppositories, or small volume microenemas, for the purpose of maintenance since these are likely to cause less discomfort to the patient. Use of microenemas in the initial stages of faecal impaction is less likely to give favourable results than use of the phosphate enemas although they can be advantageous if the individual has problems with retaining the larger volumes of fluid.

The problems which an individual with colonic constipation may experience differ from those of people with rectal constipation, in that they frequently suffer from the loss of liquid, rather than solid, stool which gives the impression that they have diarrhoea as opposed to constipation. This needs to be carefully assessed. If necessary medical staff should be encouraged to consider referring the patient for radiological examination, which will reveal faecal matter in the colon, before any interventions are commenced. The reason for the apparent presence of diarrhoea is that the faecal mass in the colon is causing a degree of obstruction to the liquid stool above it. This then begins to leak around the solid faecal matter and down to the rectum. Failure to recognize the problem of impaction with overflow can result in wholly inappropriate measures being taken which are directed towards correction of the diarrhoea serving only to exacerbate the problem.

Although the long term measures which can be taken to prevent recurrence of colonic constipation are generally similar to those required for rectal constipation, the initial management differs. Administration of rectal enemas is often ineffective in clearing the obstruction since they do not penetrate sufficiently far into the colon to reach the faecal matter. The use of large volume soap and water enemas, although uncomfortable, is one method which can stimulate colonic emptying and again these may need to be used over a period of days to ensure complete clearance. Laxatives such as senna, or sodium picosulphate, are also comparatively effective although they can cause a very dramatic bowel motion which may involve pain and discomfort for the patient coupled with a short term increase in the risk of soiling. Dietary considerations also differ somewhat for individuals suffering from colonic constipation, since there is a risk that a high fibre diet can lead to increased colonic loading particularly if the person has a delayed transit time. Excessive fibre intake under these circumstances will increase rather than decrease the risk of further episodes of constipation. Because of this it may be more effective to concentrate on efforts which are directed towards an increase in fluid intake, rather than an increase in fibre, and the long term use of stool softeners such as lactulose.

DIARRHOEA

By definition diarrhoea is considered to be the frequent passage of loose stools. When considering the relationship between diarrhoea and incontinence it is necessary to broaden this definition somewhat since the presence of loose stool in the rectum, regardless of how frequently it occurs, may lead to incontinence.

Diarrhoea may be an acute problem for an individual or it may be more chronic in its nature.

Acute diarrhoea

Generally speaking acute episodes of diarrhoea result from infection of the bowel as a consequence of food poisoning. Other than this, acute problems may be the result of an intolerance to a specific food, or drink, or may be related to anxiety provoking events. In reality any stimulus which increases bowel motility significantly, results in a decrease in transit time and hence a decrease in the amount of water which is reabsorbed and the formation of more liquid stool. Certain drugs, notably antibiotics, are also notorious for causing acute diarrhoea due to their effect on the normal bowel flora, and this should always be borne in mind when assessing a patient.

Chronic diarrhoea

Anyone who is suffering from a chronic, or recurrent, problem with diarrhoea requires full and thorough investigation since it may be related to a new growth of the bowel and may be the first symptom which a person presents with. Bowel neoplasms, whether benign or malignant, interfere with fluid absorption and normal bowel function resulting in the production of more liquid faeces. This is often accompanied by mucus and/or blood. Other chronic bowel disorders such as Crohn's disease and ulcerative colitis have a similar effect.

DIARRHOEA AND INCONTINENCE

In a healthy individual, sphincter control is often sufficient to maintain continence even in the presence of comparatively severe diarrhoea. In any individual who is debilitated, as can occur rapidly when suffering from diarrhoea, or who has a less than intact sphincter control mechanism, the ability to retain the liquid faeces in the rectum may be completely, or partially, lost leading to faecal incontinence and soiling. This is true for both chronic and acute episodes of diarrhoea and is aggravated, in the case of infective diarrhoea, by the fact that the peristaltic action of the bowel is increased as a result of irritation. This causes the faeces to be propelled into the rectum at a greater rate and with greater force than normal, causing excess strain on the sphincter which may not be able to retain the faeces. In all cases of diarrhoea it is essential to attempt to isolate the cause and a full investigation should be carried out by the medical team.

Any person who is incontinent of faeces as a result of having diarrhoea is likely to experience a greater range of problems than someone who is incontinent of formed stool, since the liquid faeces are not only more difficult to contain but are also more likely to cause skin excoriation. Initial interventions to promote continence in this situation are aimed at control of the diarrhoea by administration of prescribed anti-diarrhoeal medication, the majority of which act by slowing transit time and therefore affording a greater chance of fluid reabsorption.

Sphincter weakness

Weakness of the internal or external anal sphincters has a similar effect on an individual's ability to control faecal continence as weakness of the urinary sphincter does on the ability to maintain urinary continence. The causes of anal sphincter weakness are also broadly similar. Loss of muscle tone due to ageing, trauma or denervation are the predominant causes. The latter two may be aggravated by a history of constipation and straining to evacuate the bowel. One further cause of anal sphincter damage is that caused by repeated stretching of the sphincter as a result of sexual activity.

Mental state

As with urinary incontinence individuals who have lost the ability to discriminate what constitutes an appropriate time and place for defecation or who are unable to find the lavatory may suffer from faecal incontinence not associated with any of the above causes.

NURSING INTERVENTIONS FOR FAECAL INCONTINENCE

Once again the first step towards promoting continence for individuals who are incontinent of faeces is to establish whether they have any pattern to their incontinence. Assessment and recognition of a pattern can be carried out in exactly the same way as for urinary incontinence. One very common finding is that people will have their bowels open first thing in the morning when they are given a drink or breakfast. This is due to the gastrocolic reflex described earlier. In smokers this reflex may also be stimulated by the first cigarette of the morning, and it is not uncommon for people who stop smoking to become slightly constipated for a period of time after giving up.

Management of individuals who demonstrate a pattern of defecation and incontinence directly related to food intake may present a problem in terms of philosophy of care and feelings of 'decency'. The simplest form of containing the faeces under these circumstances is to ensure that the person is sitting on a commode, or the lavatory, when the stimulus, be it food, drink or a cigarette, is ingested. Many people find the concept of a patient sitting on the toilet while having their breakfast to be unacceptable. The alternative, however, is that the patient will be sitting in a pad filled with faeces, a situation which may be equally unacceptable. This is something which will need to be considered carefully, and in consultation with the patient and his or her carers.

If no pattern is evident then management of the problem relies on appropriate containment of the faeces.

Various factors need to be taken into consideration when considering containment. A more detailed discussion related to the range of pads and pants for the management of incontinence can be found in Chapter 9. However some mention needs to be made with specific reference to the management of faecal incontinence since there is a tendency to assume that persons who are incontinent of faeces require a very large pad or an 'all in one' nappy type aid. This is not necessarily the case and the decision on which pad should be used must be based on a full assessment of the problem. This includes consideration of the nature of the faeces (formed or diarrhoeal), the amount of faeces lost, the times at which the person is incontinent, the person's lifestyle and mobility. All of these have a bearing not only on the type of pad which is used but also on how disruptive this will be to the person's normal life.

MEDICAL MANAGEMENT OF FAECAL INCONTINENCE

The initial stages of any medical management related to faecal incontinence will normally concentrate on identification of the cause including treatment of any constipation or diarrhoea with appropriate medication. One further means of management is also available and may be advocated by some doctors. This relies on the use of anti-diarrhoeal medication, usually some form of opiate derivative such as codeine phosphate, which is administered on a regular basis in order to constipate the patient. Once constipation has been achieved the patient is then given twice weekly enemas, or occasionally suppositories, in order to evacuate the bowel (Barrett, 1992). This form of management can be very successful but it can lead to a comparatively high degree of discomfort for the patient and also carries the risk of inducing a greater level of constipation than necessary which will require more aggressive management than simply the use of phosphate enemas. Despite this it is sometimes appropriate for the benefit of both the patient and the carers to adopt this approach and it should not be discounted as an option.

Despite the fact that in reality there are fewer nursing interventions which can be utilized in order to promote continence in individuals who are incontinent of faeces, it should not be considered to be an impossible challenge. Full consideration of all the factors which can influence a person's bowel function coupled with sensible bowel management and, if necessary, containment measures will, if a positive attitude is adopted, greatly improve quality of life not just for the patient but for the carers as well.

REFERENCES AND FURTHER READING

Barrett, J. (1992) Faecal incontinence, in *Clinical Nursing Practice* (ed. B. Roe), Prentice Hall, New York.

Glanze, W. (ed.) (1986) *Mosby's Medical and Nursing Dictionary*, 2nd edn, C.V. Mosby, St. Louis.

Thomas, T., Egan, M. and Meade, T. (1985) Prevalence and implications of faecal (and double) incontinence. *British Journal of Surgery*, **72** (Suppl), 5141.

Tortora, G. and Anagnostakos, N. (1990) *Principles of Anatomy and Physiology*, 6th edn, Harper and Row, London.

Trounce, J. and Gould, D. (1990) *Clinical Pharmacology for Nurses*, 13th edn, Churchill Livingstone, Edinburgh.

Watson, J. and Royle, J. (1992) *Medical-Surgical Nursing and Related Physiology*, 4th edn, Baillière Tindall, London.

9

Other considerations

Although the previous chapters have considered a range of specific patient problems with regard to incontinence, there are also some general factors which need to be taken into consideration if a truly holistic approach to care is being adopted. These include assessment of the environmental and social factors which impinge on the individual, choice of appropriate clothing, sexual aspects related to incontinence and, very importantly, the correct choice of aids to help the person to manage the incontinence within his or her particular setting and individual lifestyle. As with all elements of assessment this process should begin on first contact with the patient. This is usually less of a problem if patients are being seen in their own homes since the assessment is not wholly reliant on verbal information from them and/or their relatives, but can also be based on direct observation of the environment. In an institutional setting, whether on a ward or in an out-patient department, it is important to establish as accurately as possible any home factors which may be relevant to the continence problem. It may be necessary to arrange for a home visit by nursing staff and the occupational therapist in order to clarify any outstanding questions and arrange for any modifications to the home which may be required.

ENVIRONMENTAL AND SOCIAL FACTORS

The range of possible areas which could be included within this section is enormous. There are, however, certain points which merit particular attention since they are comparatively general in their application and are also amenable to interventions by nursing staff, or by other health care workers at the instigation of the nursing staff.

Toilet facilities

This may seem to be a somewhat self-evident area to be considered but in reality it is rare to see any note of what facilities patients have at home recorded on their admission documentation or even on their continence assessment. Before considering alternatives the comfort and the practicalities of the existing toilet arrangements must be investigated. Factors such as lighting, warmth, the presence of grab rails or other supports, the height of the toilet itself, the availability of washing facilities and, not least, the size of the room need to be taken into consideration. All of these may have a bearing on the willingness and the ability of the individual to use the toilet both during the day and at night time.

Accessibility of the toilet is perhaps the commonest and most important problem for the majority of people suffering from incontinence and takes on particular significance for those with severe urgency and mobility problems. A large proportion of houses have a toilet either on the ground floor or on the upper floor but not usually on both. This presents problems for any individual who has difficulty with climbing or descending the stairs and the most frequent solution is the provision of a commode, or a urine bottle for men. In many cases this may, in reality, be the only practicable solution to the problem since major reconstructive works on existing properties are not only prohibitively expensive but may also be undesirable. Generally few problems are encountered by men who are able to use a urine bottle (although some of the following discussion can be applied equally to the use of urinals) but provision of a commode in isolation, without considering the range of problems which this can cause, is insufficient. Firstly there is the consideration of privacy for the person using the commode. This is likely to present more difficulties in a family setting or if the individual lives with a partner who, regardless of how long the couple has been together, may never have seen any other member of the family on the toilet. At worst this situation could lead to the incontinent person being isolated to a room of his or her own, effectively imprisoned by incontinence.

There are however certain other less dramatic steps which can be taken to help to alleviate the extent of the problem. One item which should always be provided at the same time as a commode is some form of screen. This is essential even if there are no other people living in the household since the commode is very unlikely to be used in the toilet itself and, unless individuals are prepared to have the curtains of the room in which they use the commode drawn at all times, they may be anxious about the possibility of being seen from the street while using it. Net curtains are not sufficient for this purpose.

Although lack of privacy of this nature may not have a direct bearing on a person's level of incontinence it may have a significant effect on quality of life. Despite the fact that a screen will not prevent noise and odour from reaching other people sitting in the same room, it may be sufficient to provide enough privacy to put the person using it at some degree of ease. An alternative to this is for other family members to leave the room while the commode is in use. Their willingness to do this will depend very much on the relationships that exist within the family and it may be that the individual concerned would not be prepared to impose this degree of disruption on other family members regardless of whether or not they would be happy with this arrangement. Another approach, which assumes some degree of warning of the need to void and sufficient mobility on the part of the individual, is to have the commode placed in an adjoining room which the person can reach with little difficulty. This is often the best compromise but it still requires the provision of a screen in order to prevent exposure to the windows and members of the family who may need to enter the room.

The potential problem of odour from a commode also needs to be taken into consideration since this may lead to as much embarrassment within a family setting as use of the commode in the first place. Discussion should take place with regard to this and the way in which odour can be minimized by the use of air fresheners and, if available, products which form a gel on contact with the urine which help to reduce odour and also the risk of urine spillage when the commode is being moved or emptied. This is also a useful addition to urine bottles particularly with regard to the prevention of spillage. In the absence of this, spillage from urine bottles may be prevented by use of a 'non-spill' adaptor which comprises of a rubber flutter valve which only allows passage of urine into the bottle.

Emptying of the commode in itself may present a problem

for some individuals and their families. Assessment of the ability of family members and their willingness to perform this task should be routine, accompanied by instruction as necessary in terms of infection control and the importance of keeping the commode clean and emptied immediately after use, if possible, to minimize the chance of stagnation of the urine and the subsequent increase in odour and bacterial growth. The same is equally true, if not more so, if the commode is being used for bowel elimination.

In some cases even if individuals are able to use the toilet other pressures within a family setting may cause them to experience incontinent episodes. If they require assistance to get up, or walk to the toilet, it may be difficult for them to keep asking other family members for help, particularly if they are occupied doing something else. This can lead to a situation where an individual waits for as long as possible before asking to got to the toilet and experiences some degree of leakage in consequence. This situation can also occur in institutional settings either as a result of individuals not wishing to 'bother the nurses' or sometimes due to the attitude of the nursing staff themselves when asked. A refusal or avoidable delay on the part of care staff in toileting will usually result in an episode of incontinence and very often have the rather more far reaching effect of preventing the patient from asking again and thus cause not only an increase in the number of incontinent episodes but also a decrease in the person's self-esteem. This type of behaviour on the part of care staff is unacceptable, regardless of whether it stems from laziness or ignorance, and needs to be identified and acted upon accordingly by care managers. In a home setting the reluctance may be overcome by encouraging the individual and other family members to be open about their fears and discuss the problem honestly. This may lead to a greater degree of understanding for all parties and a consequent reduction in embarrassment and anxiety.

Protection of furniture and bedding

This is a particularly important consideration since soiling of furniture is not only embarrassing for the individual who is incontinent, but it also carries with it associated problems (and costs) of cleaning and odour. The potential for the individual to become socially isolated may be increased since it is unlikely that he or she will be prepared either to invite others into their home or visit others if there is a risk of the furniture becoming wet. Needless to say providing some means of containment and protection is not a substitute for promoting continence; for most people who have undergone a programme of continence promotion this problem should be rare if it exists at all.

Leakage of urine on to furniture can occur for a number of reasons. Firstly there may be an episode of unexpected incontinence as can occur if a person forgets to self-catheterize or fails to go to the toilet at the appropriate time. Strict adherence to an individual toileting or catheterization programme should help to prevent this from occurring, but if there is any doubt the individual should be encouraged to use an appropriate pad to contain any leakage which may occur. Choice of pads, which will be addressed more fully later in the chapter, is also important since the use of ill fitting or poorly applied pads can lead to leakage round the edges and subsequent wetting of clothing and furniture. An alternative to body worn pads for the protection of furniture is the use of underpads. The major problem with these is that they are usually obtrusive and difficult to disguise. In an individual's home setting this may not cause particular difficulties but someone who has visitors, or is visiting friends or relatives, may be reluctant to use them. Regardless of the setting certain people may choose to put the pad into a cushion cover to make it more aesthetically acceptable – either on its own, or with the cushion if that is what they normally sit on.

If persistent soiling of furniture is occurring then it may be advisable, even in a home setting, to consider purchasing commercially produced chair and mattress covers specifically designed for the purpose of preventing damage from incontinence. A number of companies also manufacture chairs with impermeable covers which are more often found in institutional settings. There are some disadvantages with these, however. They are comparatively expensive and, because of the nature of their covers, they tend to lead to a greater accumulation of sweat around the buttock and groin area with a consequent increase in the risk of pressure sore formation, infection and odour. One further problem with this type of covering is that if a person is incontinent of a large amount of urine there is an increased likelihood that it will run on to the floor and soil the carpet necessitating more frequent cleaning.

CLOTHING

For many incontinent people this is a very problematic area since they feel severely restricted with regard to what they can wear. In some cases this is of course true but in the vast majority the range of clothing which can be worn by individuals with a continence problem is little different to that which can be worn by any other person. There may, however, need to be certain compromises made as to the style of clothing worn or, if possible, the management of the incontinence.

Particular difficulties may be encountered if a person wishes to wear tight trousers, skirts or dresses. In all these cases it is more likely that any external means of managing the incontinence will be apparent through the clothing. Ways in which the inconvenience from this can be minimized include use of less bulky pads, or use of a smaller volume leg drainage bag, both of which will be less obtrusive under clothing. The drawback to both of these is that they will require more frequent attention than the larger appliances but some individuals may consider that it is worth the effort in order to wear a wider range of clothes. Regardless of the use of smaller appliances it does have to be acknowledged that external management is still likely to preclude the wearing of skin tight clothing in most cases.

The other main problem area which is encountered by both sexes is if the incontinence is managed by use of an indwelling catheter. Regardless of the length of catheter used (i.e. female as opposed to male length) it is virtually impossible to hide a leg drainage bag under a pair of shorts or a very short skirt. The same problem applies to the majority of swimwear. It is possible to conceive of various contortions which could be applied to ensure that the leg bag remains invisible, however, there are only two certain ways of doing this. The first is removal of the catheter completely for the period which the person requires followed by re-insertion later. During this time the individual will need to adopt a different form of management (e.g. ISC, pads) but, assuming that the person's original need for catheterization was properly assessed and that this was the only appropriate way of managing the incontinence, alternative means are likely to prove less effective even over a short period of time and the person needs to be made aware of the potential problems associated with them. The other realistic alternative is that the closed drainage system is broken and the catheter spigoted off. This of course obviates the need for a drainage bag and in the majority of cases the individual will remain dry until the pressure within the bladder rises to the point that urine is forced out around the catheter. In order to avoid this the spigot will have to be removed and the bladder drained at appropriate time intervals which can really only be determined by practice and experience on the part of the individual. It would seem that overcoming this problem without to some extent compromising the principles of reducing infection risk in catheterized patients may be impossible. For some this compromise, although possibly not to be encouraged if one is approaching it strictly from the angle of a health professional, may be worth the increased risk in order to allow them to dress according to their wishes, at least for some of the time.

Certain problems may be encountered by individuals even if they are not overly concerned about fashion in general. Sadly the image which is often conjured up when clothing is considered in relation to incontinence is one of elderly women with split back dresses and no knickers on. This is in fact a very accurate reflection of the standard of clothing which was offered to incontinent people in institutional settings in the not too distant past. Fortunately times have changed for the better and certain companies specialize in the production of appropriate clothing for people who are incontinent. A question does remain, however, about the wearing of underwear. Although pants and knickers which give easy access for pad removal and replacement are available they do tend to be somewhat bulky in themselves and also may be unsightly. For people who are mobile and simply have difficulties in reaching the toilet in time this type of aid is wholly inappropriate and it may well be that they would in reality prefer not to wear any knickers at all since the time it takes to remove them may make the difference between being wet and managing to use the toilet. This again emphasizes the need for involvement of individuals themselves and allowing them the freedom to make choices about their own care and management.

In many cases it will be possible to make minor modifications to existing clothing in order to make removal easier. This is essential for those whose main problem is a degree of urgency and also for those who have reduced mobility and/or manual dexterity. For all these people the speed at which they can remove or undo their clothing may be crucial to the main-tenance of continence. The simplest and most common modifi-cation is the use of Velcro in place of buttons or zips which provides not only a secure closure when required, but also the potential for rapid opening. One problem which is en-countered particularly by men is the size of the handle on the zip of trouser flies. These are often very small and difficult to grasp and may delay the opening of the flies for a significant length of time. This can be overcome by insertion of a small safety pin or paper clip through the hole in the handle which gives a larger item to grip whilst still being small enough to hide discreetly in the flap of the fly.

One last but extremely important consideration in relation to clothing is the ease with which it can be washed and dried and the facilities which the individual has for this. Even with the best management systems some leakage and soiling of clothing is likely to occur and this will necessitate extra laundry. This may create a huge burden for people who have limited facilities for laundering and drying their clothes and for those who have restricted incomes, particularly since there is no statutory re-quirement for a service to be provided by local authorities. One consequence of this is that soiled clothing may be stored until there is sufficient to make up a washing machine load. This leads to a potential odour problem and also rotting of the fabric neither of which are desirable. Extra benefits may be available for some people and, if financial difficulties are identified as a problem, referral to a social worker should be considered in consultation with the patient.

SEX AND INCONTINENCE

The link between incontinence and the genital area inevitably raises questions related directly to the sexual act and the ex-pression of the individual's sexuality. Unfortunately these questions are often left unasked and, if they are asked, sometimes unanswered, as a result of embarrassment on the part of the individual and in some cases on the part of the staff as well. This is, however, an area which deserves consideration and attention from nursing staff since problems related to sexuality may have a profound effect on the ability of individuals to form or maintain relationships and hence on their general health.

In order to understand fully the effect that incontinence may have on a person's sexuality it is first important to consider the scope of sexuality in general terms. Definitions of sexuality differ somewhat but the majority are in full agreement that it extends beyond the mere genital aspects of sex (although these are obviously important) to include far broader concepts. Lion (1982) suggests that sexuality extends to cover '. . . all those aspects of the human being that relate to being boy or girl, woman or man, and is an entity subject to lifelong dynamic change. Sexuality reflects our human character not solely our genital nature'. Bearing this in mind it is apparent that how people choose to express their sexuality may be highly individualized and it would be as mistaken to make assumptions in this area as it would be in any other aspect of care. Coupled with this is the idea that sexuality is not a static concept and that it may change, not only as a result of physical and psychological maturation, but also in response to an altered state of health.

Since sex and sexuality remain comparatively private and personal areas of discussion it is likely that an individual experiencing sexual difficulties will be reluctant to approach nursing staff about them. Because of this it is important that nurses are not only aware of the fact that patients may wish to discuss the subject, but are also sufficiently comfortable in themselves to talk openly and freely about sex without displaying any signs of reluctance or embarrassment and, when necessary, will be prepared to initiate discussion on the topic. The potential problems related to the physical and psychosocial aspects of sexuality are not easily categorized, and there will inevitably be some degree of overlap, with physical aspects often initiating a predominantly psychological response, and psychological aspects manifesting themselves as a physical problem. As with all other aspects of caring for incontinent people, individual needs must be assessed and action taken accordingly.

In real terms it may not be possible for nurses themselves to undertake the sort of psycho-sexual counselling which is required in order to help patients come to terms with problems which are predominantly psychological in origin. Such patients are likely to need the help of a counsellor trained in this field. Despite this nurses still have a significant role to play – not only as referral agents to trained counsellors but also in relation to the physical problems which may be associated with in- continence. Since this is not a book on sex therapy or psycho- sexual counselling, the following sections will address some of the potential problems which may be associated with in- continence. This is not intended to be an exhaustive list, but merely a selection of problems which may be amenable to nursing intervention.

Physical problems associated with incontinence and sex

Genital soreness   This problem is not restricted to the field of sexuality and sexual contact and may present difficulties for anyone who suffers from incontinence. It is however of parti- cular significance if any genital contact is to take place. Sources of soreness may vary, the commonest being direct irritation resulting from the continued presence of urine or faeces around the genital area. This should be avoidable by appropriate management of the incontinence which serves to minimize the length of time which the urine/faeces is in contact with the skin and by washing the groin area and changing pads or pants as soon as they become soiled. The possibility of infection should also be excluded since this may be masked by the presence of excoriation due to chemical irritation.

Another source of skin soreness is the use of ill fitting pads or pants which leads to friction. This is further exacerbated by the presence of urine and it should be easily solved by supply- ing aids of the correct size for the patient. The other aids which may lead to skin problems are the adhesive urinary sheaths. Some individuals are allergic to the adhesive supplied with the sheaths under which circumstances there is likely to be a discrete band of soreness where the adhesive has been in contact with the skin. Alternatives such as an inflatable condom sheath should be considered, or sheaths which are designed to be secured by external means. Under no circumstances should an attempt be made to secure the sheath to the penis using tape wrapped around the sheath. This may not only lead to transient discomfort for the patient but may also cause damage to the penile circulation.

Leakage of urine during sexual contact   This can be a problem for both sexes, although it is more common in females, particularly during intercourse. It can be avoided, or at least minimized, by trying to ensure an empty bladder prior to sexual activity. Some individuals may need to empty their bladder at some point during sex, and it is helpful for them if they can estimate when this will be needed rather than experiencing leakage. Leakage may be due to direct pressure on the bladder as a result of the position adopted during sex. Experimentation with different positions may help to minimize the problem, and this can be discussed with the individuals concerned.

In all cases of leakage couples are likely to feel more at ease if the bed, or other surface, is protected with a waterproof covering. Care may need to be taken in the choice of protection since any covering which rustles, or is particularly mobile (as is the case with plastic undersheets), could be very distracting for a couple who are trying to have intimate sexual contact.

Odour   Genital odour can present a problem in any relationship, but is more likely to be present if an individual is incontinent. Dependent on the extent of the odour problem it may only be apparent if the couple are having oral sex and in most cases it should be avoidable by careful washing of the genital area, particularly prior to sex. If this still does not solve the problem the possibility of infection in the groin area (often fungal in origin) should be excluded and treated appropriately. Under these circumstances the odour is often related to the presence of the infective organism, and therefore more difficult to remove by superficial washing of the area.

Impotence   In physiological terms this is a problem which should not be directly linked to incontinence unless the incontinence results from damage to the nerve pathways which

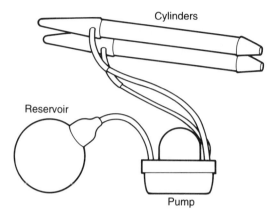

Figure 9.1 Example of an erectile prosthesis.

are responsible for initiating an erection. In a number of patients the impotence may be psychosomatic in origin and the individual or couple may need referral to a specialist counsellor. If the cause of the impotence is physical in origin various options are available to the patient. These range from papaverine injection to surgical implantation of erectile prostheses (Figure 9.1), and again referral to the appropriate specialist should be made.

Presence of an indwelling urinary catheter Contrary to popular belief the presence of a catheter does not remove the possibility of full sexual expression, regardless of the sex of the catheterized individual. Men with indwelling urinary catheters can bend the catheter down the shaft of the penis, leaving a small loop at the meatus to avoid the risk of trauma. The catheter can then be secured to the penile shaft with a small piece of adhesive tape, taking care not to encircle the penis with it. Securing the catheter in this way minimizes the risk of traction. This can also be achieved, to a lesser extent, by the use of a contraceptive sheath applied once the catheter has been positioned along the shaft of the penis. Some individuals may choose to utilize both methods (Figure 9.2). If a sheath is not being used, or if it is unlubricated, some form of additional lubrication may be necessary both for comfort, and to reduce friction on the catheter. It should be remembered that despite

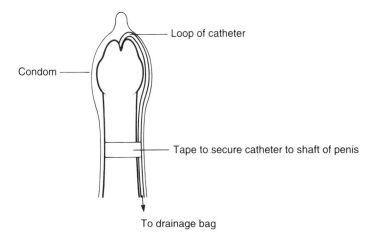

Condom

Loop of catheter

Tape to secure catheter to shaft of penis

To drainage bag

Figure 9.2 Position of catheter and sheath in preparation for penetrative sexual intercourse.

the fact that there is a catheter *in situ* there may still be the possibility that viable spermatozoa will be emitted from the urethra, and contraceptive measures should be taken as appropriate to the needs of the individuals concerned.

In the case of a woman with a catheter *in situ* it is possible to tape the catheter to the abdomen or the thigh in order to ensure that it is as unobtrusive as possible. For both men and women care needs to be taken with the drainage bag to keep it out of the way during sex since there is a possibility of urinary reflux up the drainage tube or, in extreme circumstances, the bag could split if undue pressure is applied to it. Couples may choose to disconnect the bag altogether during sex and spigot the catheter. Apart from the obvious risk of increased infection rates resulting from breaking the closed drainage system, there is also a risk of urine leaking around the catheter if the volume in the bladder becomes too great. This may not only cause discomfort for the individual concerned, but could also be a distraction from the enjoyment of the occasion.

Individuals who are able to catheterize themselves, or have a partner or carer who is able to perform the catheterization, may choose to remove the catheter before sex and replace it afterwards. This again carries a slightly increased risk of infection which should be borne in mind when choosing how to manage the catheter in relation to sex. One other point which should be considered is that, if there is an infected discharge around the catheter, unprotected penetrative (particularly vaginal) sex should be avoided in order to minimize the risk of spreading the infection, and medical advice should be sought in order to obtain appropriate treatment.

AIDS FOR THE MANAGEMENT OF INCONTINENCE

This is an area where there is great potential for confusion both on the part of health care professionals and incontinent people themselves. There are literally thousands of different aids on the market ranging from pads to penile clamps. For this reason it is important to consider some general points which should be borne in mind when choosing an aid with a patient. These are as follows.

Comfort

This element can be considered to be of prime importance in an aid since if the person experiences discomfort when using a pad or appliance they are unlikely to continue to use it for any length of time, regardless of how effective it is. This will lead to an increase in problems for the patient and may also result in an increase in the number of incontinent episodes. Discomfort results from various factors such as the size of the appliance, how tightly or loosely it fits, the length of time for which it is worn and, not least, the material from which it is made. Since comfort levels are obviously a highly subjective concept and unique to the individual it is essential that they are discussed with the patient who should be made aware that there are alternative aids available if the one being tried proves unsuitable. Psychological comfort must also be considered and it is not acceptable to try to force an individual to use a pad which, for any reason whatever, causes that individual distress.

Size and absorbency

This predominantly applies to incontinence pads, however, size may also be an important factor to consider when choosing items such as urine drainage bags. As mentioned above, the size of an appliance can make a tremendous difference to what type of clothes an individual feels able to wear. The choice of which pad to use is often determined by which pads are readily available and how much urine or faeces is lost. In the former case availability has probably been decided by a supplies department rather than by a nurse or continence adviser. Although it may be difficult at times to obtain alternatives to the stock items it is not sufficient to accept this without question if the nurse considers that a different pad would be of more benefit to the patient. If the volume of urine lost is to be used as a criterion then pad absorbency, rather than size alone, needs to be considered since, dependent on the manufacture of the pad, some smaller pads may well absorb sufficient urine to keep the patient dry and prevent leakage. Details of pad absorbency can usually be obtained from the manufacturers or from the *Directory of Continence and Toiletting Aids* (Association for Continence Advice, 1992). In general terms the smaller the pad which can be used the better since this is likely to be less uncomfortable for the patient and also less obtrusive under clothing. In general terms it should be unnecessary to use a pad which holds more than 300–400 ml (i.e. the equivalent of a full void) since the pad should be changed when wet in order to avoid the problems of skin excoriation and sore formation. The only exception to this may be at night or if the individual specifically wishes the pad to be changed less frequently.

Many pads are supplied with elasticated knickers to hold them in place and, although these may be less aesthetically acceptable to the person, it has been found that they reduce the amount of leakage around the pad when compared with using ordinary underwear.

Cost

This is often the deciding factor for many people when choosing which pads and appliances to carry in stock. In reality the cheapest pad is not always the most cost effective and careful evaluation of pads should be carried out prior to purchase. The other factor which needs to be borne in mind in relation to this is that proper assessment of individuals should result in the most appropriate pad being supplied to meet their needs and that this may well be a cheaper pad than is available from stock since these are, in many cases, a larger size of pad than most people require.

TYPES OF AID AVAILABLE

Aids for women

When compared with the number of aids which are available for the management of urinary incontinence in the male there are pitifully few aids available for women. The majority of female incontinence is managed solely by the use of pads. Other than this there are the aids which have been described in Chapter 5 for the management of stress incontinence, but in real terms little else. This is an area which merits further research and development.

Aids for men

Penile sheaths There are a large number of different penile sheaths which are available from manufacturers, the majority of which rely on the use of adhesive to attach the sheath firmly to the penis. The main variation between them is that some sheaths are 'one-piece' and have the adhesive applied to the inner surface of the sheath itself and others are 'two-piece' and utilize an adhesive strip to hold the sheath in place. In the final analysis there is very little to choose between these two systems for the majority of people and the choice of which system to use is very much dependent upon individual preference. In both cases certain principles apply and must be taken into consideration prior to application of the sheath since incorrect application can lead to leakage and the risk of the sheath falling off, both of which are unpleasant for the patient. The first and probably most important condition to consider before application of a urinary sheath is the size of the penis itself. Urinary sheaths are totally unsuitable for use on very short and retracted penises since there is not enough length in the penile shaft to allow for sufficient contact with the adhesive. Penile diameter is less crucial than length in this respect, but is significant when it comes to choosing the correct size of sheath and where possible some sort of sizing guide should be used. Application of a sheath which is too large will result in leakage and increased risk of the sheath falling off, whilst use of a sheath which is too small will cause pain and discomfort to the patient with the ultimate risk of compromising the penile blood supply. One practice which is particularly dangerous, and still takes place from time to time, is trying to hold the sheath in place with adhesive tape which is not supplied for the purpose at the base of the penis around the outside of the sheath. Because there is generally little or no elasticity to this type of tape penile blood supply can be affected significantly.

Removal of the sheath is effected in most cases by a rolling action up the penis and care should be taken to ensure that no pubic hair is stuck to the tape since this is painful for the patient when pulled. One way of avoiding pubic hair becoming incorporated into the sheath is to use a sheet of card or a tissue around the base of the penis to hold the hair out of the way during the application stage. Most manufacturers recommend that sheaths should be changed every 24 hours and that the skin should be cleansed and checked for any signs of breakdown or allergy to the adhesive. If a person is experiencing skin problems as a result of the adhesive, use of the sheath should be discontinued and alternative management considered until the skin has healed. One alternative is to use a sheath which does not rely on adhesive to anchor it in place. Two main forms are available, those which have an elasticated band, which is supplied with the sheaths and can be placed round the sheath to hold it in place, and those which have an inflatable cuff at the base of the sheath which when inflated holds the sheath in place. The latter form tend to be considerably more expensive than the adhesive kind, but they are re-useable and may prove to be more economical in the long term for some patients.

Aids for men with a retracted penis As mentioned above, sheaths are unsuitable for men who have a retracted or particularly short penis and they will require other forms of management. The simplest aid available for men who are unsuitable for a sheath is the retracted penis pouch, a device which is similar in concept to an ostomy bag. It consists of a

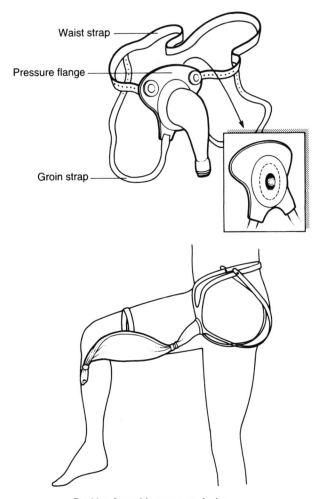

Position for pubic pressure device

Figure 9.3 Pubic pressure device.

bag which can be stuck to the pubic area, following a shave, using the integral adhesive backing through which the penis can be passed. Following this the hole in the backing is positioned directly over the point where the penis retracts so that any urine which is lost is contained. This can then be drained off into a normal drainage bag.

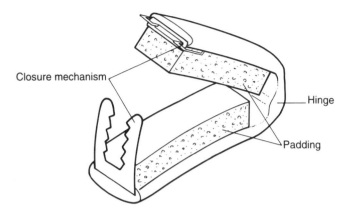

Figure 9.4 Penile clamp.

The other aid which is most commonly used for a man with a retracted penis is the pubic pressure device (Figure 9.3). The combined arrangement of the belt and the flange serve to put pressure around the base of the penis which in turn forces it out through the opening in the flange. Covering this opening is the removable bag or cone which can be drained in the normal way. These appliances need to be sized for individual patients and are almost tailor made in some cases; one complaint regarding them is that they are somewhat bulky. This, coupled with the initial cost of the appliance, may deter some people from considering their use.

Penile clamps The penile clamp is an occlusive device which is placed around the penis and closed (Figure 9.4). Although popular with some individuals as a short term measure to provide occlusion to urinary leakage, it does have obvious potential disadvantages with regard to compromising the penile blood supply. Penile clamps should therefore only be used with great care and a full understanding on the part of the patient of the risks involved.

Drip collectors Often referred to as dribble pouches these can be of great use to a man who only has slight dribbling incontinence and should also be considered for post-prostatectomy patients who frequently experience a short term dribbling incontinence. The pouches are normally attached to the inside of standard or, in some cases, specially supplied underpants by the use of an adhesive strip. The penis can then be placed into the pouch and any leakage, up to approximately 100 ml for some products, is contained. Since the penis is enclosed within the pouch, and therefore in contact with the urine, it is particularly important to ensure that proper attention is paid to skin care and if possible to use a product which retains the urine behind a non-return membrane.

RE-USEABLE PRODUCTS

With an increased emphasis on environmental considerations, cost effectiveness and acceptability of the product to the consumer there is a huge potential for the use of washable pads and pants. Consideration should, however, be given to the hidden costs of these products such as laundering, and a full assessment of these should be made (Philp, Cottenden and Ledger, 1993). Although the re-useable underpads which are available have a comparatively large capacity the washable underwear does tend to have a significantly lower absorbency than pulp or gel filled body worn pads and may therefore be unsuitable for people who lose large volumes of urine in one void. They should not be discounted, however, since they may be suitable for people who have frequent loss of smaller volumes of urine. They are usually a good deal less bulky than the pulp pads and it is therefore easier to carry a spare pair around. There is obviously no problem with disposal of soiled pads and the majority also look more like 'normal' underwear than pants designed to hold a disposable pad. Most people find them more acceptable to hang on the washing line. Drying of re-usable products may present problems for some people and again this needs to be considered when recommending products for client use (Norris, Cottenden and Ledger, 1993).

In reality there is no simple formula for choosing which aid to use for the management of incontinence. Probably the most important factor is a willingness to actually take the time to investigate what is available and to try to match this with the needs of the individual patients as identified by the assessment process.

REFERENCES AND FURTHER READING

Association for Continence Advice (1992) *Directory of Continence and Toiletting Aids*, Association for Continence Advice, London.

Clancy, B. (1989) No more guesswork! Choosing incontinence products. *The Professional Nurse*, June, 455–6.

Lion, E. (ed.) (1982) *Human Sexuality in Nursing Process*, John Wiley, New York.

Norris, C., Cottenden, A. and Ledger, D. (1993) Underpad overview. *Nursing Times*, **89**(21), 65–8.

Philp, J., Cottenden, A. and Ledger, D. (1993) Well disposed? *Nursing Times*, **89**(16), 65–8.

10

Starting a programme

The emphasis throughout this book has been, very firmly, on the positive aspects of continence promotion. The most significant factor affecting the success or otherwise of a programme of continence promotion, both on the level of the individual patient and at an institutional level, is the degree of motivation on the part of all those concerned. It cannot be over stressed, however, that the approach adopted initially by nursing staff not only influences how well their care (and that of their colleagues) is delivered but also how patients and their carers perceive the problem and its eventual outcome. It is therefore important to consider what factors serve to motivate, and also de-motivate, staff, patients and carers.

FACTORS AFFECTING MOTIVATION

As mentioned in Chapter 1, certain problems may be encountered when attempting to interest staff in the field of continence promotion due to its comparatively low-tech and unglamorous image. Because of this, careful planning needs to be made prior to starting any continence promotion programme and changes in clinical practice. Ideally a team leader or facilitator needs to be identified from the ward or community team. One of the first prerequisites for success is that whoever is chosen (or preferably puts themselves forward) to 'head up' any moves towards commencing a continence promotion programme, has an overt belief in the benefits of it. Such people are not always easy to find, neither are they necessarily the most senior individuals in the nursing team. In this context the most important factor is that they will be able to motivate other members of staff and also be seen to be credible in what they are doing and saying. This can only be achieved through study, experience and a very high level of enthusiasm for the task since it is likely that there will be some resistance, be it active or passive, from other members of the team, certainly in the initial stages of a programme.

Once the decision has been made to implement a programme and a facilitator (or team leader) has been identified, the next stage is to provide at least a basic level of information and education for the other members of the care team. This achieves three main aims. Firstly it helps to involve other team members and gives the opportunity for them to share their knowledge and views on the subject. Secondly it helps to ensure that there is a degree of continuity of approach to care from all the members of the team. The third and most important result of this initial input is that there is likely to be a higher level of co-operation, if not enthusiasm at this stage, from work colleagues who will be expected to participate in the implementation of the programme. If possible the continence adviser should be involved from the start of the planning stage in order to provide specialist input.

Although the exact nature of the information which is given at these initial meetings will vary, a broad sequence of events needs to be followed. Firstly it is important to determine the views, experiences and current knowledge of the team members in order to maximize the existing potential and to build on it. This part of the process will also help to identify any individuals who would be willing to play a more active role in setting up the programme. The second stage of the process is to sell the concept of continence promotion to any team members who may have doubts about it. This is of course easier said than done and it is useful at this point in the proceedings to enrol the help of the continence adviser, if one is available, and also any staff from other areas who have been successful in implementing a programme. Following this an 'educational' package needs to be provided for the staff to give them a sound knowledge base from which to work.

Once the staff have been introduced to the topic it is then possible to begin to put the theory into practice. Again this is often easier said than done and one of the common mistakes which is made is to attempt to implement the plan on too large a scale. This creates difficulties in monitoring the success of the programme and also increases the potential for staff to become disillusioned if the number of patients who fail to respond rapidly to the interventions is high. A more reasonable approach which is likely to provide positive feedback for the staff, and therefore increase motivation, is to be selective in the early stages about which patients are started on the programme. Initially, at least, it is best to concentrate on patients who are likely to achieve continence, or an improvement in their condition, comparatively fast. This demonstrates clearly to all those involved in their care that continence promotion really does work in practice. This approach does not mean that the level of care for other patients who are incontinent will be decreased and they can be included in the programme when appropriate.

Although the most appropriate person to facilitate this process is probably a nurse it is important not to exclude other members of the multidisciplinary team, particularly the doctors. These may be the most difficult group to involve in the programme, regardless of whether they are in general practice or hospital care, since they frequently see the problem of incontinence as being solely the domain of the nurses. Gaining the support of a consultant or the senior partner in a practice will usually help to increase the motivation and interest of their junior colleagues which is essential if a truly holistic approach to the patient is to be achieved.

Once a programme has been established it is important to maintain the impetus and the enthusiasm which has been built up amongst the staff. One of the most successful ways in which this can be done is to encourage attendance on courses and study days related to continence promotion, coupled ideally with the instigation of research projects directly related to the area in which they are working. The latter serves not only to increase local interest in the topic but will also contribute to the wealth of knowledge which already exists on the subject. One particular area which lends itself well to research of this nature is comparative trials of incontinence aids such as pads and pants, a field where there is always room for more indepth and objective information.

EDUCATION

Education and staff development is essential if continence promotion is to remain at the forefront of people's minds and become embodied as part of the philosophy of care. It should not be restricted however to the qualified or permanent staff in the area. With the increase in the number of health care assistants and clinical support workers greater emphasis will need to be placed on their development and skills than may have been apparent in the past with nursing auxilliaries. This is particularly important since they will, in a large number of clinical areas, be responsible for delivering a high proportion of the hands-on care which the patients receive.

This need for education is equal, if not greater, amongst student nurses. The development of Diploma in Higher Education (Nursing) courses and a greater number of degree pathways for nurses has led to a greatly increased emphasis on the use of nursing research to inform clinical practice. If the concept of continence promotion is to be taken seriously within this academic framework this emphasis will need to be reflected not only in the classroom setting but also in the clinical areas where the students are gaining their experience. One way of ensuring that this occurs is the use of standards coupled with an appropriate rationale based on other people's research, but probably more effective and meaningful is, as mentioned earlier, on-going research within the clinical area itself, carried out by staff who are working directly with the patients on a day to day basis. This is not, of course, a substitute for appropriate and informed tuition within a classroom. Work carried out by the King's Fund (1983) suggested that at that time there was some input to pre-registration nursing courses with regard to the management of incontinence with a minimal amount of time devoted to the promotion of continence. One of the reasons for this was doubtless that the teachers themselves had had little or no formal teaching on the subject and had therefore little to pass on to their students. Although the emphasis within the clinical areas may have changed to give a comparatively high profile to the concept of continence promotion it has to be remembered that the students of 1983 may well be the nurse teachers of today. With the number of changes which have taken place in nursing – and nurse education in particular – over the past 10 years, it is quite possible that they have failed to update or educate themselves with regard to continence promotion and that the only knowledge they have is based on what they themselves received as students during their training. This is unlikely to be adequate for the needs of today's students and it is incumbent on the teachers (as it is on all nurses) to ensure that their knowledge base and competence is up to date in order for them to provide appropriate information and support for their students and for qualified staff in the clinical areas. This may mean that the teachers themselves need to attend courses on the promotion of continence since it is no longer adequate for the topic to be regarded as one which can be taught by anyone. Teachers in the field need to be committed to the subject and, as with any other subject, keep themselves constantly updated.

Apart from the obvious need for nurses to have a sound knowledge base to inform their clinical practice in terms of the actual interventions they carry out, they also need knowledge in order to provide patient education. Because of the somewhat entrenched attitude that may be encountered when discussing incontinence and continence promotion, it is important for nursing staff who are involved in an area where a continence promotion programme is being carried out to have a sound knowledge of why they are doing things and not simply what to do. This will not only ensure that correct information is given to the patients but also that the nurses will, rightly, be perceived by the patients as competent. This will encourage the development of a greater trust in the nurses' ability on the part of the patients and their carers, and a consequent increase in motivation and compliance with any individualized programme which is proposed by them.

BUDGETARY IMPLICATIONS

In real terms there are very few long term cost implications involved in promoting continence. The highest initial costs will be related primarily to staff training. These costs can be kept to a minimum by adopting the approach advocated above of having one individual who can act as a 'key trainer' for the other staff in the area. This does not of course obviate the need for time to be set aside for all the staff involved to receive training on the subject and it should be possible to include this as part of any on-going staff development programmes which are taking place in the clinical area.

In the longer term it is likely that the implementation of a continence promotion programme will result in considerable financial and resource savings to the area as a result of the following factors. Firstly fewer patients will require pads, secondly the pads which are used will be the most cost effective and thirdly there will be lower laundry costs. It is difficult to predict exactly what level of saving will be achieved in any given area, but even in the absence of figures it is important to persuade the budget holder for the area that continence promotion will inevitably result in some saving both in material resources and nursing time. The support of the budget holder will greatly enhance the chances of the programme's success in the early stages and, with the increased emphasis on financial savings which has developed over the past few years, will also help to ensure continued support for the programme in the future.

The final and perhaps most important group of people who need to be totally involved in the planning and implementation of the programme are the patients themselves and their carers. Regardless of how enthusiastic the nursing staff are, it is the individuals affected by the problem who have the most profound need for hope. Without this hope, motivation levels are likely to be low and the chances of successful continence promotion will be reduced. Patient education, delivered at a comprehensible level, will go some way towards developing an appreciation of what can be achieved, but perhaps the most important factor is the joint planning of care with the patient and the setting of realistic goals within a patient centred framework. This can only be achieved if the staff involved with the patients have a sound knowledge base themselves which further emphasizes the need for continued staff development. Another approach to consider is the development of a patient and carer support/social group. The exact nature and aims of this will of course vary dependent on the needs of the area and the group. It does, however, have the potential to be used as an information giving group and also to increase the confidence of those individuals who may have become isolated as a result of their incontinence. This form of group may also be helpful to carers who again can use it to share information and for mutual support.

The success of a continence promotion programme should be evaluated at regular intervals. This evaluation needs to be based on a wide range of factors and not simply the financial aspects of the endeavour. One of the first areas that needs to be evaluated is the degree of patient satisfaction with the service. Ideally there should be some measure of this prior to embarking on the project so that a comparison can be made. This not only serves to measure the success of the programme but can also help to direct the programme in the early stages since it will give some indication of what the patients themselves feel is required of the service. Use of properly designed questionnaires which can be filled in by patients or their carers should yield the information which is required. These questionnaires will need careful analysis in order to draw meaningful conclusions from them. The same information gathering exercise can be carried out with the staff who are to be involved in the programme since their level of satisfaction and acceptance of the project will ultimately determine its future.

More objective measurements related to costs, including the number of pads used and any changes in laundry expenses and other peripheral items, will also need to be made prior to the inception of the project in order to provide figures for analysis. Other data which should be collected if the overall picture is to be complete includes the number of patients who are incontinent and the number of incontinent episodes which occurred, again prior to and after the start of the programme. This full evaluation process will, of course, not be possible in all settings since it takes time to carry out, and there may also be difficulties in obtaining the necessary data. Regardless of this some form of evaluation or audit process must be included as part of the initial planning for the programme, if for no other reason than to provide evidence to staff involved in it, and to the budget holders and managers, that it was worth the effort – and the cost. A more far reaching effect of carrying out a full evaluation is that the information will be of use to other areas that are considering setting up a programme, and in certain circumstances elements of it may even be suitable for publication in the nursing press. This not only disseminates the information but, if the evaluation has been carried out in a systematic manner and has been presented appropriately, also broadens the research base of continence promotion.

Although setting up a continence promotion programme may initially appear to be a somewhat daunting task, the rewards for both patients and staff once it is established should far outweigh the problems which are encountered along the way. The key factor for success is motivation and determination that it will work. In real terms it will probably be impossible to attain the ideal (whatever that may be) but any small step towards it can make a significant difference to everyone concerned.

As mentioned in Chapter 1, nurses are in an ideal position to inspire and co-ordinate continence work within the framework of the multidisciplinary team and as such should be encouraged and supported in that role by all members of the team. This includes support from nurse managers who must have the confidence in the ability of their staff to plan and initiate changes in clinical practice within their specialist area. Most importantly this support must go further than simply allowing the change to take place. It must include financial and human resources to enable the project to succeed. Only by doing this will quality patient care in the field of continence promotion be achieved and the negative attitudes of the past be dispelled.

REFERENCES AND FURTHER READING

King's Fund (1983) *Action on Incontinence*, King's Fund, London.
Meek, D., Thorne, P. and Luker, A. (1989) Support groups for older women. *Nursing Times*, **85**(46), 71–3.
Rooney, V. (1984) A team for continence. *Journal of District Nursing*, April, 6 and 11.
White, H. (1990) Playing a central role. *Nursing Times*, **86**(16), 73–5.

Appendix A

Abnormalities of urine

Urine testing by the use of observation and dipstick tests is a procedure carried out on an almost daily basis by nursing staff. Since this procedure is frequently used as a primary screening technique it is important that nurses have a knowledge of the meaning of the test results and what constitute abnormal readings. Correct interpretation and reporting of the results may not only lead to an earlier diagnosis and hence treatment for the patient but also to a financial saving, since it may obviate the need for further analysis of the urine in the laboratory. Observation of the urine is a comparatively straightforward but nonetheless important activity. The exact nature and the range of substances which can be detected using test strips vary from manufacturer to manufacturer and this section will give an outline of the substances most commonly tested for, and how their presence in urine may be interpreted. It is important to stress that accurate testing using this method relies on following the manufacturers' instructions particularly in relation to reading the results at specific times which may be necessary for quantitative analysis. Fresh urine should always be used for the test.

OBSERVATION OF THE URINE

Colour

The colour of normal urine varies between a very light yellow to a dark amber. Normally this is dependent on the concentration of the urine and diet. Certain diseases may also have an effect on this. Consistently light coloured urine may be the result of excessive urine production, as would occur in diabetes mellitus and diabetes insipidus, whereas production of very dark urine may be indicative of some form of hepatic or biliary disease and the presence of large amounts of urobilinogen. The other commonest form of urinary discoloration is that caused by the presence of blood which may present as frank blood or, more frequently, as a mild pink discoloration. Drug therapy, dyes used in radiological examination and diet should all be considered as potential causes of abnormal urinary discoloration and excluded prior to considering any more sinister causes.

Turbidity and the presence of casts

Normally urine is clear and transparent in appearance. At times it may appear cloudy as a result of the precipitation of phosphates and carbonates which become insoluble in alkaline urine. This cause of cloudiness, which does not constitute an abnormality, can be excluded by acidifying the urine (normally done by the addition of acetic acid) which should cause the urine to become clear. The main cause of abnormal urinary turbidity is the presence of pus cells resulting from infection.

Urinary casts are also responsible for causing turbidity. These consist of cells and cellular debris from the distal collecting tubules. They are indicative of inflammatory or degenerative changes in the tubules. The presence of clearly visible strings or specks of matter in the urine is often indicative of infection, but may in some cases be the result of contamination of the specimen with other secretions produced by the genitourinary tract. This is most common in men where there may be residual seminal fluid in the urinary tract which is excreted on urination.

Odour

It is difficult to define exactly what constitutes an abnormal or offensive odour. The smell of urine can be affected by a large number of factors, most related to concentration and diet. If left standing all urine will begin to smell ammoniacal as the result of bacterial action. This smell should not be present in freshly voided urine and could be indicative of infection. Foul smelling urine is almost always indicative of infection and is also comparatively easy to recognize. Again diet and drug therapy should be considered as possible sources of 'abnormal' odours from urine.

Specific gravity (S.G.)

This is determined by the relative proportions of dissolved solids in the urine and is therefore extremely variable since it is dependent on the concentration of the urine which is being produced. Single measurements of S.G. are, therefore, comparatively meaningless and it is only when there is a consistent deviation from the normal range (1.010–1.025) that underlying pathology should be considered.

A consistently low S.G. means that there is either an excessively large volume of urine being produced by the kidneys as occurs in diabetes insipidus and, it must be remembered, in patients undergoing diuretic therapy, or as a result of diseases such as glomerulonephritis where the ability of the kidney to concentrate urine is impaired.

A consistently high S.G. may result from uncontrolled diabetes mellitus where there is a high proportion of sugar dissolved in the urine, or in conditions such as congestive cardiac failure which lead to oliguria and fluid retention. It is also indicative of chronic dehydration.

If the S.G. remains unchanged it may still be indicative of impaired renal function, since it suggests that the kidney is unable either to dilute or concentrate the urine.

pH

This again is a very variable measurement because of the role of the kidneys in regulating blood pH which results in any changes being reflected in the urinary pH. Normal values range between 4.8–8.5 although readings outside this range are not necessarily indicative of any particular pathology. In general terms a consistently low pH may be associated with starvation, dehydration and diabetes mellitus, whilst a consistently high pH will accompany urinary tract infection.

ABNORMAL URINARY CONSTITUENTS

Leukocytes

These will be found in the urine of patients who are suffering from inflammatory conditions of the urinary tract such as cystitis and urethritis and may or may not be accompanied by bacteriuria. In the absence of bacteriuria other causes should be investigated since the presence of leukocytes can always be considered to be abnormal. In women particular care must be taken to ensure that the specimen has not been contaminated by vaginal secretions which will lead to a false positive reading.

Nitrites

The presence of nitrites in the urine can be detected by some of the test sticks available on the market. This is a particularly useful test since a positive result is indicative of bacterial activity in the urine and hence urinary tract infection. An early morning urine specimen is the ideal sample for this test but failing this urine which has been in the bladder for at least four hours may be used.

Protein

The presence of protein in the urine can always be considered to be abnormal, although it may result from non-pathological sources. These include orthostatic proteinuria and proteinuria following physical exertion. The commonest pathological cause is upper urinary tract infection.

Glucose

Classically the presence of glucose in the urine is considered to be indicative of diabetes mellitus and is frequently the first indication which is given of the condition when routine urinalysis is performed. There are, however, various other causes and glucose may be found in the urine following a meal particularly rich in carbohydrates, during pregnancy, in those with a low renal threshold for glucose and in certain individuals with renal damage.

Ketones

Ketones, or ketone bodies as they are sometimes referred to, are produced as a result of fat metabolism. This occurs primarily in two situations. The first is when there is insufficient glucose within the body to provide the energy required for normal metabolic processes to take place. Starvation, weight reducing diets and cases of severe vomiting will cause this. In the absence of any of these ketonuria is indicative of a disturbed glucose metabolism as occurs in diabetes mellitus. The presence of ketones in this group of patients should always be treated as significant, particularly if glucose is also present, since high levels of ketones in the blood lead to ketoacidosis, coma and the potential for central nervous system damage.

Urobilinogen

This is produced from bilirubin in the gut as a result of bacterial action. Under normal circumstances all urobilinogen that is produced is reabsorbed and broken down by the liver. If excessive urobilinogen is produced as occurs in the case of increased haemolysis, infection of the biliary tract and certain gastrointestinal conditions (e.g. severe constipation leading to a much decreased transit time) the liver may be unable to metabolize the higher blood levels and it is then excreted in the urine. The other situation in which this can occur is acute or chronic inflammation of the liver resulting from infection or other conditions such as cirrhosis or carcinoma.

Bilirubin

This is an abnormal constituent of urine and is only found in cases where the serum bilirubin levels are grossly elevated. This can occur in cases of acute and chronic hepatitis, cirrhosis and biliary obstruction. It is not present in cases of prehepatic jaundice.

Blood

The majority of test strips now available differentiate between haematuria, the presence of intact red blood cells, and haemoglobinuria, the presence of free haemoglobin resulting from the breakdown of red blood cells. Haematuria can be further divided into gross haematuria, where the urine is discoloured by the presence of blood, and microhaematuria, where the urine appears normal but red blood cells can be detected by microscopy or chemical tests. Haematuria may be indicative of a number of conditions including the following:

- urinary tract infection
- trauma
- renal or bladder calculi
- tumours of the urinary tract
- glomerulo- and pyelonephritis
- hypertension.

The presence of haemoglobinuria may be the result of severe haemolytic anaemias, poisoning, burns, systemic infections and physical exertion.

In some circumstances both haematuria and haemoglobinuria may be detected. This may be the result of haemolysis taking place in the specimen and the test should be repeated using a fresh sample.

Appendix B

Useful addresses

Age Concern (England)
Astral House, 1268 London Road, Norbury, London SW16 4EJ.
Tel 081-679 8000.

Association for Continence Advice
The Basement, 2 Doughty Street, London WC1N 2PH.
Tel 071-404 6821.

Association for Spina Bifida and Hydrocephalus
ASBAH House, 42 Park Road, Peterborough PE1 2UQ.
Tel 0733 555988.

Disabled Living Foundation
380–384 Harrow Road, London W9 2HU.
Tel 071-289 6111.

Enuresis Resource and Information Centre (ERIC)
65 St Michael's Hill, Bristol, BS2 8DZ.
Tel 0272 264920.

Multiple Sclerosis Society
(Headquarters), 25 Effie Road, Fulham, London SW6 1EE.
Tel 071-736 6267.

National Action on Incontinence
4 St Pancras Way, London NW1 0PE.
Tel 081-892 6898.

Sexual and Personal Relations of the Disabled (SPOD)
286 Camden Road, London N7 0BJ.
Tel 071-607 8851.

Spinal Injuries Association
Newpoint House, 76 St James's Lane, London N10 3DF.
   Tel 071-444 2121.

The Continence Foundation
2 Doughty Street, London WC1N 2PH.
   Tel 071-404 6875.

Telephone helpline

Continence Service
Tel 091-213 0051.

Index